SEXPERTISE

SEXPERTISE

Real Answers
to Real Questions
About Sex

DR. ROBIN SAWYER

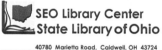

SIMON SPOTLIGHT ENTERTAINMENT

New York London Toronto Sydney

SSE

SIMON SPOTLIGHT ENTERTAINMENT
A Division of Simon & Schuster, Inc.
1230 Avenue of the Americas
New York, New York 10020

First Simon Spotlight Entertainment trade paperback edition
April 2008

SIMON SPOTLIGHT ENTERTAINMENT and colophon are
trademarks of Simon & Schuster, Inc.

For information about special discounts for bulk purchases,
please contact Simon & Schuster Special Sales at
1-800-456-6798 or business@simonandschuster.com

Designed by C. Linda Dingler

Manufactured in the United States of America

10 9 8 7 6 5 4 3 2 1

Library of Congress Cataloging-in-Publication Data

Sawyer, Robin G.
     Sexpertise : real answers to real questions about sex / by
Robin Sawyer.
          p. cm.
     ISBN-13: 978-1-4169-5346-3 (pbk.)
     ISBN-10:   1-4169-5346-9 (pbk.)
     1. Sex instruction—Popular works. 2. Sex—Popular works. I.
Title.
HQ31.S285 2008
613.9071—dc22   2007049537

To Anne, Katherine, Emily, Meg, Gillian, and all my students at the University of Maryland

Contents

The Communication Basics: Let's Hook Up or Whatever   27

Part Two: Everything You Really Should Know About Sex

Before Sex, During Sex, and After Sex   55

Before Sex   56

D
R

R
O
B
I
N

S
A
W
Y
E
R

During Sex 95

After Sex 119

Part Three: The Other Stuff

It's Just a Little Rash: Sexually Transmitted Infections (STIs) 131

The Plague of the Century: HIV/AIDS   155

Gay, Bi, or Hopelessly Confused: Alternate Sexual Expression   167

I Seem to Have a Little Problem: Sexual Dysfunction 179

D
R

R
O
B
I
N

S
A
W
Y
E
R

He Wants to Put What Where? Atypical Sexual Behavior   197

Part Four: Our Sexual History

Foreword

Pizza Boy . . . where are you now?

Approximately twenty-two years ago, I was teaching my human sexuality course for the first time in the BioPsychology Building at the University of Maryland to an auditorium of five-hundred students. The topic was sexual response, and I was exposing my students for the first time to a very graphic film that showed—well—how men and women respond sexually. Now, I'm bound to assume that most of my students have seen porn films but there is always a rather nervous tension that develops when five-hundred strangers sit in a dark room watching a Swedish man frantically tugging at his extremely swollen member. On the one hand (no pun intended), students know this is a class and they need to concentrate and examine the film from an academic perspective. However, on a more fundamental level, all the researchers in lab coats taking notes and ECG readings in the world can't alter the fact that what they're observing is a big Scandinavian dude whacking off, right there on the screen in front of them. Hence, a little anxiety.

As this segment of the film reached its climax (sorry, I can't help myself), the tension in the room was palpable, particularly as Sven had progressed to using two hands and was tugging so violently it seemed that his unfortunate penis would be painfully disconnected from his body. At this precise moment, a sharp rap on the door, accompanied by a cry of "Pizza man!" heralded the arrival of a warm Italian pie and a moment that would forever change the life of the person I now fondly remember as Pizza Boy.

As the door flew open I can only imagine what terror the young man must have felt when instead of a hungry customer, he discovered a darkened room with five hundred shadowy figures all turned to focus on his face. That would have been bad enough, but at this very moment of shock, Sven's prolific on-screen ejaculation was accompanied by a prolonged moan that bounced off the walls of the auditorium.

I have no idea what Pizza Boy was thinking. Perhaps he thought that he'd unwittingly stumbled upon a coven of sex addicts undergoing some type of carnal initiation ritual (with, of course, full student government funding). Well, whatever was actually racing through his mind at that moment, Pizza Boy knew he had to get away. Literally throwing the boxed pie up in the air, Pizza Boy screamed, "Oh shit!" and dashed away into the night, in my imagination, forever scarred.

Wherever you are today, Pizza Boy, I hope you can forgive me—and Sven!

Introduction

Does the world really need another book on sex? Aren't you sure you know all about sex? Well, maybe not *all* about sex, but as much as the average person? In fact, given the amount of material on sexuality freely available in magazines, on cable television, and on the Internet, does anyone really need additional information? You might think not, but after spending twenty-two years teaching a university-level human sexuality course, I've come to the conclusion that despite claims to the contrary, most people really know very little about human sexuality.

This lack of knowledge is ironic considering today's highly sexualized world in which we live, compared to the monochrome days of the fifties or even the fondly remembered days of the swinging sixties. Even baby boomers, who grew up in the sixties replete with Jimi

Hendrix, dope, booze, protest marches, and free love (until, of course, we all caught an infection and worked out that nothing was really "free") didn't live in such a sexually charged world.

I often joke with my students that if sex were an Olympic sport, then the United States would be the clear winner. Every time I make this statement to a class the same ritual occurs. My students (the males in particular) hoot, high-five, and pump their fists in a frenzy of celebration at American sexual prowess. I can only imagine their thoughts turning to huge penises, delay of ejaculation lasting for days, and Olympic judges holding up perfect "10"s for a sexual performance that brings the roaring crowd to its feet. Imagine my students' disappointment when I tell them the gold medal would be awarded for having the highest teen pregnancy rate, the highest sexually transmitted disease rates, and the highest proportion of HIV/AIDS of any Western industrialized nation.

This is truly a generation of performers. I like to say that today's generation is the Nike generation—they "Just Do It!" Unfortunately, most people's focus is on the action of performing without really knowing much about the facts of what they're doing.

I've definitely seen my share of the more sexually active men—you know the type, the ones who've had their fair share, your share, and everyone else's share of the spoils and think they know everything about sex. But over the years, I've actually found an inverse relationship between the amount of experience a man claims and his sexual IQ. It's as if a man's brain matter has oozed out along with copious amounts of semen. Maybe that's where the phrase "screwing your brains out" comes from.

As to whether men or women know more about sex, the answer is clear. Women consistently know *as much* about men's sexuality as men, and *more* about their own than men. This makes perfect sense to me; if a man can't even ask directions to the mall, how will he ever be able to ask where the clitoris is? This also explains why my classes are 60 percent women and 40 percent men. Women are more comfortable admitting they don't know something and asking questions. But in fact, both sexes are in need of some help. Let's get one thing very clear:

There are no stupid questions in sex.

Quite often the very individuals who are ridiculing someone for asking a "dumb question" are actually straining to hear the answer themselves, too embarrassed to admit they don't know.

Given the abject lack of sex education currently occurring in most schools and homes, it's no accident that so many Americans reach early adulthood with their sexual experience vastly outweighing their meaningful sexual knowledge. It's my hope that *Sexpertise* will become a valuable resource for anyone who reads it. You can read it cover to cover or use it as a resource by identifying topics that are of interest to you. Sections will follow the logical progression of our all too familiar courting and mating rituals—from looking, to talking, to touching, to doing, to consequences . . . good and bad. *Sexpertise* will allow you to get answers to questions you might consider foolish and might correct some information that you thought you knew but really didn't.

I've also included two in-depth sections on contraception and sexually transmitted infections. When you're armed with knowledge, unintended pregnancy and contracting an infection are preventable. *Sexpertise* also includes a section on what many of you at first glance will consider an oxymoron—sexuality and aging. Well, it's not—you just don't know it yet. One day you'll be fifty years old, or even sixty, and will be really happy you read this book. For now, this section may make you feel a little odd around your parents or grandparents, but you'll get over it. The best may be yet to come!

Throughout *Sexpertise*, please note that laughing about sex, and most importantly, laughing at yourself, is an absolute requirement. If you can't laugh about sex, you'll eventually be paying out big dollars for sex therapy. So enjoy the read, and for goodness sakes, smile—it's only sex!

PART ONE

The Basics

The Physical Basics: From
Tubes to Testes

Despite supposedly having received mandated sex education in public middle and high school, most Americans actually know very little about reproductive anatomy. Some people blame this ignorance on a conservative movement that pushes the mantra of "abstinence-only-until-marriage" education (and I use the term "education" loosely), but even the opponents of sex education grudgingly allow a little anatomy to slide into the curriculum. However, the more likely culprits of this ignorance are the two most common, but all too dubious sources we go to for information on sex: peers and the media.

Friends telling friends about sex has a warm ring to it, but let's be fair, these are the same friends who routinely have one-night stands, get too drunk to use contraceptives, use grape jelly because they're out of K-Y, and refuse to use condoms because they'd never have sex with someone who had an infection. The media is also an endless source of useless information, particularly prime-time television, where the message is loud and clear—only extremely attractive people actually have sex, and the rest of us must live vicariously through who and what we see on our television screens. And the sex we see is usually spontaneous, contraception optional (let's not ruin the moment), with negative consequences never amounting to anything more than fleeting regret. Oh, if only life could be so forgiving.

This section of the book will deal with who has what parts and what function those parts serve. This section will not be divided into male parts and female parts as I feel strongly that we should all know much more about each other.

Is man's largest sexual organ the penis?

Fortunately not. The largest sexual organ of all humans is not located between our legs but between our ears—it's the brain. Our large brain distinguishes humans from every other species on Earth, and to a great extent, controls our sexual response. (Although some people think a man's brain is jammed into his penis until he reaches the age of thirty, by which time the brain manages to crawl up into his cranium, despite all too common bouts of suction in the op-posite direction.)

How do humans compare to other primates with regard to the penis?

Compared to our closest relatives, other primates, a human's penis is much larger, both in length and girth. The average human male's penis even trumps that of a huge, hairy gorilla. This fact should make some of us feel a whole lot better!

Does size matter?

For vaginal intercourse, anything around 2.5 inches can get the job done because a woman has no nerve endings on the inner part of the vagina, and most sexual sensation is derived from the clitoris, which is external. There is little or no established infor-mation on the implications of penis size for either anal or oral sex. What should be remembered is that the stimulus for most of our sexual response is psychologi-cally influenced. So if someone happens to have a predetermined affinity for a particularly large penis, then his or her response to a smaller member might prove less than satisfying.

Does girth matter?

Great question. Girth may actually be *more* important than length. We've just stated that the vagina has its majority of nerve endings in the outer part of the organ, so perhaps length is less of an issue. In addition, don't forget, the legendary G-spot, which is located on the upper vaginal wall and is stimulated primarily by pressure that would be more likely to occur if the penis was thicker. Remember, the vagina is an elastic organ that can expand to allow a baby to pass through during childbirth and yet also hold a relatively slim tampon during menstruation—the implications for adapting to various penis widths are obvious.

Is it possible for a penis to be too large?

From a male perspective, this may sound impossible, but once you get past the testosterone and the ridiculous visual imagery of Stallion Boy, having an incredibly large penis could be a problem. Some heterosexual women have complained that a large penis can be very painful in certain sexual positions to say nothing of an obvious gag reflex problem when performing oral sex. So, yes, too big can be too much.

What is the normal size of a penis?

"Anything two inches less than mine" is the typical male's answer, and he's sticking to it! There are several studies in existence, but the problems surrounding an accurate measurement of the penis via self-reporting are all too obvious. In nearly every penis-measurement survey where men self-report the data, the reported average size of the penis is larger than the result of studies done through observation and direct measurement. What a surprise! For a study that involves getting a boner in a lab setting, wouldn't the volunteers be men who have larger penises? Isn't it unlikely that Mr. Microphallus will show up to publicly display his shortfall?

Alfred Kinsey had a collection of thirty-five hundred sets of penile measurements. The longest authenticated measurement of an erect penis according to his records was 10.5 inches, with the average erect length being 6.2 inches. More recently, in an attempt to address this eternal question, the American Urological Association established a guideline that suggests the average penis is 3.5 inches long when flaccid and grows to an average of 5.1 inches when erect. (I can predict the sighs of relief and gasps of elation as some of you arrive at this point of the book to realize you have more than you need.) The circumference is an average 3.9 inches, which expands to 4.9 inches when erect. The learned doctors of genitalia made the day for many a man when they announced that the "normal" length for a penis would be anything above 2.8 inches when erect. This figure takes into account a wide range of lengths in addition to the minimum length anticipated to provide satisfactory sexual intercourse.

Is it true that you can tell how big a man's penis is by the size of his shoes?

Don't be ridiculous. But I'd like to think you *can* tell a man's penis size by the car he drives. The bigger the car, the smaller the penis—a big sorry to those damn Hummer drivers. I, naturally, drive a Mini Cooper. I really do.

Is it true that certain races or ethnic groups have larger penises?

Another interesting question. I must preface my answer by stating that it's based on urban legend rather than fact. There are very few studies that can answer this question accurately, and again, researchers run into methodological problems. One study looked at condom breakage rates, making the assumption that the ethnic group with the most breakages must therefore have the biggest penises. But what if that particular group had a disproportionate number of men who were lousy condom users, and the condom breakage had nothing to do with penis size? The World Health Organization (WHO) recom-

mends the following *width* sizes for condoms distrib-
uted geographically: 5.3 centimeters (cm) wide for
Africa, 5.2 cm wide for Europe, and 4.9 cm wide for
Asia. (No numbers in evidence for the Americas.) The
differences in size are statistically very small and support the concept that while there will be an obvious
range of size within each group, there is no evidence
to support the idea that one ethnic group has a substantially larger penis size than any other.

Does penis circumcision make any difference during sex?

A growing body of evidence has gradually eroded
the belief that male circumcision is a necessary procedure, and despite earlier concerns over various
health issues, the consensus seems to be that circumcision, at least for medical reasons, is unnecessary. In the United States, rates of infant circumcision
ranged between 80–90 percent during the 1970s
but that proportion has since decreased to around
60 percent. Other countries reflect much lower per-
centages: Canada 35, Australia 13, England 6 and
Scandinavian countries around 2 percent.

There's no research to suggest that sexual satisfaction with or without a foreskin is any different for men
or women. In fact, when an uncircumcised man's
penis is erect, the foreskin is drawn back and his penis
looks exactly the same as the penis of a circumcised
man. Many people circumcise their male infants for

religious reasons, but that reason aside, in a world where men are obsessed with penis size, I'm always surprised that we would take the trouble to trim off a few centimeters. Who knows when you might be glad of that little bit extra?

OK, you say it doesn't matter, but do women prefer circumcised penises?

What's best, a snail wearing a helmet or a snake wearing a sweater? I've heard preferences for both the circumcised and uncircumcised penis. Some women prefer the more streamlined look of the penis minus the foreskin while others laud the excitement of the "natural" penis, suggesting that with the foreskin there's more going on and more to play with. The bottom line is, it's not what you have but what you do with it.

Does all semen taste the same?

Although there is no definitive research on this issue, subjectively speaking there is a theory that the types of food a man eats can affect the taste of his semen. If the theory (and it is only a theory) holds true, it seems that vegans will have the most pleasant-tasting semen, as fruits seem to be the least offensive food, while meats can be less desirable. Here are a few examples of how different foods *might* affect taste:

- Semen can be sweetened by drinking lots of pineapple juice or eating bananas or papayas.
- Red meat can make the semen taste more acidic.
- Alcohol or coffee can make semen taste more bitter.
- Garlic, onions—both have a high sulfur content that can make your semen taste bitter.
- Cinnamon reportedly sweetens the taste of semen.

Is semen high in calories?

A typical amount of ejaculate is about one teaspoon, although the actual volume can vary, mainly influenced by the last time the man ejaculated. Semen is not high in calories as 90 percent is made up of water, with other ingredients including proteins, carbohydrate enzymes, cholesterol, and trace amounts of iron and zinc. The simple sugars that provide the sperm with food on their long journey amount to about five or six calories. Oral sex will not make you fat!

Is semen high in protein?

The amount of protein in semen is very small, probably no more than about six milligrams. One urban legend suggested that semen contained as much protein as a pork chop—hardly. A small pork chop would typically contain as much as twenty-four grams of protein, dwarfing the amount found in semen.

Is it true that swallowing semen reduces the risk of breast and ovarian cancers?

Yes, and swallowing also increases your IQ, makes your hair shine, and guarantees that you'll win a gold medal in GULLIBILITY. The initial purveyor (and his fellow distributors) of this "seminal" information had to be a man. He gets points for the sheer balls of using an outrageous line like that. And who knows, maybe it's even worked once. Why not? I mean, come on, he's doing you a favor. By providing you his semen (free of charge)—that can only be extracted from his body through fellatio—he's actually protecting you from cancer. What a guy. There could be a Nobel prize in this for him. And the long-awaited answer to this question would be a profound *no*.

What's the hymen and what does it do?

The hymen is a membrane that covers the opening to the vagina, and its presence has been traditionally associated with virginity. In "days of old" checking the intact condition of the hymen to confirm a woman's chastity and purity was not an unusual occurrence. Like other body parts, the hymen is variable in nature, meaning in some women it is thicker and more strongly attached, in others very flimsy and easily torn, and in some, is nonexistent. Its purpose, in an evolutionary sense, was probably to provide some rudimentary form of protection to the opening of the vagina. However, realistically, the hymen would certainly provide no protection from a marauding penis and so has little practical function.

Can you tell if a woman is a virgin?

The presence or absence of a hymen, a membrane that covers the opening to the vagina, doesn't prove whether or not a woman has had sex before. Despite being a historical symbol of chastity, many hymens have broken and disintegrated long before a young woman has intercourse for the first time. However, in some societies where female virginity is especially highly prized, the practice of hymen reconstruction has evolved. The hymen reconstruction surgeon takes a very sheer piece of animal membrane, lightly sutures it across the opening of the vagina, and voilà, she's a virgin—again. (This is your first example of how women are much smarter about sex than men.)

A man thinks he knows three things about a female's loss of virginity: there will be pressure (because of the hymen); there will be bleeding; and, inevitably, there will be pain.

When the wedding night arrives, "Jack the lad" leaps into his connubial bed only too anxious to deflower his young bride and rightfully claim, to use the male vernacular, her cherry. Makes him sound like a damn fruit picker, but that's guys for you. Intercourse begins and, yes, there's some pressure as the new hymen is tested; there will inevitably be a small amount of blood as the sutures give way, and the bride doesn't have to be Meryl Streep to emit some convincing wails of pain. So there we have it . . . pressure, blood, pain, another maiden deflowered, a man's honor satisfied. It doesn't get any better than that. There is no easy way to accurately determine whether or not a woman is a virgin.

What is the clitoris, and how will I know it when I see it?

Ah, the age-old question—and if you think this question is difficult, wait until we try locating the G-spot. An important point for men to understand is that just as all penises don't look the same, clitorises can also look slightly different from one woman to another. The clitoris is a small, flesh-colored projection located at the apex of the labia minora (inner vaginal lips), and in most cases you can't actually see the clitoral glans (the length or body of the clitoris) as it's often hidden beneath some skin called the clitoral hood. When a woman becomes sexually aroused her clitoris becomes engorged with blood and is more visibly erect. The clitoris is unique to the female in that its role is purely to provide sexual stimulation. Men may argue that their penis does the same thing, but they would be forgetting that occasional urination thing. Because the clitoris is made up of some of the same erectile tissue found in the penis, it is capable of erection when stimulated. Though much smaller than the penis, the clitoris has twice the number of nerve endings, and in fact has a higher concentration of nerves than anywhere else on the body.

Are most women shaving their pubic hair these days?

For the past few years more and more young women are shaving off their pubic hair. How did this trend begin? I've no idea, but what has become apparent is that many young women seem to almost equate pubic hair with uncleanliness, to the point where they make a face when you even mention *that* hair! These women are a far cry from their predecessors in the sixties where hair everywhere was de rigueur. Today's trend of being a slave to the Brazilian wax provides an alarmingly prepubescent look that I suppose provides great protection against crabs—nowhere for those little darlings to congregate!

Do women prefer men to shave too?

Through my research I've established that many women prefer a man who, in female-speak, is "well groomed." Because of this burgeoning perception that pubic hair is messy and unwanted, many women do not want a male whose crotch looks like a hairy monkey's rear end. Some men have imitated their female counterparts and removed all offending hair, but many have simply trimmed back the pubes hoping, undoubtedly, to give off an air of sophisticated, well-manicured genital urbanity. A Web site extolling the virtues of a shaven male body exists (*www.shaveeverywhere.com*), although the site—owned by Philips—might have as much to do with marketing their body-grooming razor as offering a commentary on the wonders of a hairless body.

Does the anus have a G-spot?

What you're referring to is the male's prostate gland. The gland lies about three or four inches into the anus, on the other side of the anal wall. This little gland is what every lucky man over forty years of age gets to have his doctor rub once a year as part of a search for lumps and possible prostate cancer. Men who have experienced this magical moment have described the sensation as a combination of wanting to urinate and ejaculate at the same time. Let's just say some men are a little unsettled by the whole procedure. Having said that, many men also enjoy incorporating a little prostate massage into sexual play; hence the notion that the anus might have a G-spot.

Does everyone masturbate?

Certainly the old joke for males is that 95 percent of men reported being masturbators and the other 5 percent lied! For women, the estimates are somewhat lower. The most telling feature of Kinsey's data on masturbation was men's obsession with appearing "normal." The men in the study were asked to report how often they masturbated and how often they thought most men masturbated. Whatever number the male reported for his own masturbation, the perceived norm was always a few times more. So for a man who reported masturbating three times a week, the perceived average was five, but for the man who masturbated a hundred times weekly, the perceived average was 105! Examining how often people masturbate, a 2006 survey of American 21–49-year-olds commissioned by *Esquire* and *Marie Claire* magazines reported that on average men masturbated 4.9 times weekly versus 2.8 times for women. I guess men must have more time on their hands!

Why do people masturbate?

There are any number of different reasons why people masturbate: curiosity, pleasure, boredom, stress reduction, response to sexual stimulation, and sometimes as a substitute for an absent partner. The idea that *most* people masturbate because they don't have a current or available sexual partner is actually a myth. In fact, individuals who have regular sexual intercourse tend to masturbate as much or more than people who have no one. Masturbation tends to be more of a complement to sexual intercourse rather than a substitute. Most males in particular tend to continue the habit (vocation?) even while in sexual relationships.

Is it possible to masturbate too much?

Many adolescent males routinely test the outer limits of masturbatory endurance with Mother Nature reining them in before cardiac arrest occurs. Some individuals do lapse into a habitual pattern, seemingly unable to stop themselves from almost constant self-stimulation. While working in a college clinic I spoke with a male student who was masturbating about six to eight times daily and was upset because his penis seemed to be losing its responsiveness (no shit!). To heighten the feeling, he had taken to rubbing raw alcohol on his penis, turning his unfortunate member into a rather eye-catching pound of ground beef. Obviously, this young man's behavior was a little extreme and his immediate discomfort was due more to the rubbing alcohol than the rubbing. But if any habitual activity gets in the way of your day job (or your penis more closely resembles tonight's dinner), then I think we can safely say you're probably overdoing it!

Are men who masturbate more likely to prematurely ejaculate?

Nothing about the act of masturbation will cause a man to prematurely ejaculate. However, under circumstances where a younger male is constantly rushing to complete his masturbatory activities quickly—perhaps because his mother may walk into the bathroom, or his father may catch him penis and *Playboy* in hand, this behavior pattern could be transferred to sexual intercourse, at least initially. The focus on rushing would be the culprit in this case, not the masturbation.

What's all this about prostate cancer and can I do anything to prevent it?

There has been a great deal of recent publicity about prostate cancer and this disease has become one of the most common forms of cancer in American men. Men's prostate glands typically grow in size as they age, and in some cases the growth is cancerous. Many nutritionists recommend eating more low-fat foods or adding supplements like saw palmetto and zinc to your diets, but all that is very boring. The best news of all comes from an Australian study. Researchers found that men who masturbated several times a week, particularly during their late teens and twenties, were less likely to develop prostate cancer than men who kept their hands in their pockets. Now,

I know that the average young man is already on a strict masturbatory regimen, but this study makes it official. You have to do it for the good of your health; it's doctor's orders.

If I have a vasectomy, will I ejaculate anything?

When a vasectomy is performed, the two vessels (vas deferens) that transport sperm to the ejaculatory duct are cut, so that sperm cannot get into the male's semen. So, the answer is, men who have had vasectomies will still ejaculate semen; it will simply not contain sperm. The volume of semen is made up in the following proportions: nearly 70 percent seminal vesicle fluid, nearly 30 percent prostate fluid, and less than 1 percent is sperm. If two guys (one of whom had received a vasectomy) masturbated, when they ejaculated, it would be impossible to determine which one had received the vasectomy just by looking at the semen with the naked eye. Now, if we got out a microscope and looked for some "swimmers," that would be a different story.

My boyfriend's penis seems to curve to one side when he's hard. Is that weird?

Many men have a penis that curves slightly to the right or left when erect. As long as the curve isn't too great, insertion shouldn't be a problem. Some men have a condition called Peyronie's disease which results in an extremely curved penis and could make insertion a huge problem. If you suspect that a problem exists, always consult a medical practitioner.

Is it normal that my girlfriend's breasts are different sizes?

It's very common for women to have slightly different breasts with regard to size and appearance. Breasts, like many other body parts, don't come in designer sets with identical precision. We just think they do after seeing so many perfect supermodels, whose slight bodily discrepancies have been carefully airbrushed away. Guess what? It's not unusual for a man to have slightly different-sized testicles too. I don't think anybody really cares about that either.

Is there any truth to the blue balls rumor, or is this an urban legend?

Ah, blue balls, the old male excuse to justify an absolute need for sexual intercourse, the inference being that if a man didn't have sex with his partner, his testicles would be so backed up with unused sperm that they would literally turn blue, and according to many a desperate suitor, quite possibly explode. I have no evidence to suggest that any young women have actually fallen for such a preposterous line, as even the most innocent of teens surely realized that a couple of very quick flicks of the wrist would have released the young man's genital tensions. There is of course a grain of truth to this theory in that if a male has an erection for some time, he will inevitably feel a buildup of pressure as his prostate fluid, seminal vesicle fluid, and sperm prepare for ejaculation. He may indeed feel an aching in his penis and testicles. But again, to remedy this problem would take only seconds, and even in the absence of such a release there is no documentation that any man's testicles have ever turned blue, far less exploded.

Do women experience the same "blue balls" feeling?

Absolutely. If a woman is sexually aroused for some time without achieving an orgasm, she will experience what we just described for men. This uncomfortable frustration in women has not been acknowledged in the same way it has for men, so no fancy name has been developed. I think it only fair to give this condition a name, so we'll call it "blue clit." Given men's proclivity for being unable to last twenty-four hours without some form of sexual release, *any* form of sexual release, it's my belief that there are thousands more cases of blue clit than there are of blue balls. It's all a matter of perspective.

Does too much testicular heat decrease sperm production?

Testicles are located outside of the body to optimize sperm development. A man's scrotal temperature is about 2–3° C lower than internal body temperatures, and sperm production requires these lower temperatures. Some men have taken this information to an extreme by sitting in very hot baths in an attempt to create their own method of contraception. Although evidence exists that sitting in a bath of hot water for thirty minutes can in some cases decrease sperm production for a few weeks, sitting in your hot tub or sauna is *not* recommended as an effective method of contraception. Tight clothing and underwear that draw the testes up close to the body may also contribute to decreased sperm production, spawning the briefs versus boxers argument. Undoubtedly, some rock stars from the eighties must have suffered from decreased sperm production as they insisted on wearing pants so tight you could actually tell their religion!

Can smoking marijuana affect a man's sperm production?

There is clear evidence that smoking marijuana on a daily basis can decrease a man's sperm production, although his sperm count will usually return to a normal range once the smoking ends or becomes less frequent. In addition to sperm production, research suggests that sperm function, namely sperms' ability to swim, can also be negatively affected by chronic marijuana use. Again, becoming a chronic pothead is not recommended as a means of contraception.

Is it true that the average man's sperm count has decreased over the past fifty years?

More than one research study has confirmed that over the past thirty years both the quantity and quality of sperm have decreased in men during this period. Research has shown that while the volume of semen has remained constant or declined slightly, the concentration of sperm has decreased significantly. Reasons for the decline are debatable but include the rise of environmental pollution, hormone presence in foods, and alcohol and drug use.

One useful factoid: If you're a woman who is trying to get pregnant, go to Finland. A recent study of sperm count conducted in three European countries revealed that the Finns have got it going on! Finnish men had a higher sperm count than men from Great Britain or Denmark, in addition to boasting a higher overall volume of semen.

Can sex count as exercise or be used for any type of athletic training?

If you're asking if sex will keep you as healthy and in shape as working out, unfortunately the answer is no. Although a vigorous bout of sweaty sex will get your heart pumping and muscles working, and *Cosmo* and *Elle* would have you believe that half an hour's sex can burn anywhere from fifty to two hundred calories, you shouldn't give up your training routine just yet.

Let's look at this the other way around. Will an effective workout regimen possibly make sex better? You bet! Working on cardiovascular fitness, stretching, and muscle strengthening will all contribute to a better sex life. Heart health will ensure efficient blood flow to the genital area, which is essential for a man's erection and a woman's vaginal lubrication; and good muscle tone will obviously help with flexibility and agility. Your early-morning workout routine may not be as much fun as sex, but not only will it make you healthier, it might just improve the quality of your sex.

Is sex good for your physical health?

Trying to prove that sex improves or worsens your physical health is almost impossible, but there are a few studies to suggest that it can't hurt! A recent Welsh study suggested that men who had sex twice a week or more experienced half as many heart attacks after a ten-year period, compared with men who had sex less than once a month. An interesting Scottish study also linked frequency of intercourse in married men to greater longevity, and additional recent studies seem to hint that more frequent ejaculation (2–3 times weekly) might reduce a man's risk for developing prostate cancer. There is also some evidence that orgasms can help alleviate women's menstrual cramping and substantially increase their pain threshold, while another study suggests, somewhat incredibly, that women who perform oral sex and swallow their partners' semen have a reduced risk for developing preeclampsia, a dangerously high blood-pressure condition that can occur during pregnancy. That particular finding seems, dare I say it, hard to swallow.

Can sex help my mental health?

Absolutely. Most psychologists would argue that sexual intercourse helps with mental health on many levels. Closeness and intimacy with another person help develop a sense of security and well-being, and during sex the brain releases dopamine and norepinephrine, two neurotransmitters that create a feeling of euphoria. Researchers have described how female orgasms boost levels of estrogen, which can help better their moods, and the production of a hormone called oxytocin that promotes feelings of intimacy increases to five times its normal level at climax. Let's face it; having sex can put you in a great mood.

The Communication Basics:
Let's Hook Up
or Whatever

In 1984, when I was teaching my human sexuality course for the first time, I was rudely introduced to the abject failure of the male to truly appreciate the strength and power of language. I was chatting with students during a class break, when an incredibly muscular student approached me. Although he wasn't wearing a team jersey, he clearly looked like a middle linebacker. Ignoring the other students waiting to talk to me, No-Neck yelled, "Doc, I need to talk to you. I'm having problems with my bitch!"

Although I knew the odds were against it, I had a momentary hopeful flash that maybe this oversized

young man was having difficulty with his golden retriever. I searched the faces of the other students who
had witnessed the question, but they were rapidly melt-
ing back into the larger student body as if fearing they
too might be called upon to provide the young man
with advice of a canine nature. "It's my bitch, Doc.
She won't do what I tell her. How am I supposed to
handle her?" I won't bore you with the details of my
rather shaken reply, but suffice it to say that my recommendation of improved communication, beginning
with dropping the term "bitch," was met with less than
enthusiasm.

Although this incident occurred nearly twenty-five
years ago, I'm constantly reminded how words can
create extremely emotive and powerful responses,
particularly words traditionally associated with sex and
intimacy. In addition, as words develop, evolve, and
change over time, their meaning often becomes ambiguous, adding to the already confusing world of sexual communication.

Has sex changed our vocabulary?

Definitely. Remember that bird in the farmyard
that wakes all the animals each morning? What's
it called? A rooster? Well, in the old days the word
for that bird was "cock," not rooster, but you see the
problem there, don't you? So you can start to understand how sexuality can influence and actually
change the English language.

Nursery rhymes that include the word haystack ("Little Boy Blue come blow your horn" etc.) have changed the original term, which was not hay*stack* but hay*cock*. Personally, I'd have been more concerned with Little Boy Blue blowing his own horn than the haycock, but that's just me. Either way, "cock" was out.

When I was of the age when you discover the power of words—particularly the "dirty" words—I would absolutely howl with delight when my father, who was carving a roast chicken for our Sunday lunch, asked me, "Do you want a leg or a breast?" What hormone-laden young boy wouldn't want a breast? The terms, "dark meat" and "white meat" were created as a response to some cultures' hypersensitivity about certain body parts.

To make very sure we never have to say the word "breast" in connection with a human female, the somewhat ridiculous term "bosom" was coined. I could never work out if each breast was a bosom or if it was a collective term for both. A fear of and discomfort with sexuality absolutely affects the language we use.

Why are we so uncomfortable with sex-related words and language?

It's all about socialization. Most of us were brought up employing absurd euphemisms for both body parts and bodily functions rather than correct anatomical terms. The unfortunate result of this approach is that most people feel uncomfortable using or even hearing correct terminology in public.

I'm a professional sex man, so when my children were born I vowed to teach them the correct terms. In our house, a penis was a penis and a vagina was a vagina. This doesn't mean that our daughters ran around the house chanting a mantra of "Penis, penis, penis." They just used the appropriate term when necessary.

Everything was fine until our daughters were old enough to be exposed to the outside world. And that's when trouble started. Our eldest daughter, Katherine, was about four years old, sitting in a supermarket grocery cart as we were waiting to check out. A long line of shoppers were patiently and silently waiting as the unsuspecting male cashier went about his business. Suddenly Katherine shattered the silence by pointing at the cashier and screaming, "He's a man! He has a penis!" Heads swiveled 'round, there were audible gasps, and the cashier's eyes bulged in his head as he visibly shrank behind the register. I was fairly tempted to step back and ask, "Whose kid is this?"

Katherine picked up on the crowd's shocked reaction and looked at me as if to say, "What's the deal? He's a guy, good chance he has a penis." Right then and there I comforted Katherine and told her that she was fine and everyone else was screwed up, although I had to retract that statement when she became a teenager, for reasons that will be apparent to every parent of a self-absorbed, narcissistic adolescent, but you see my point. People are weird about language.

What does "hooking up" mean?

You tell me! A contemporary sexual lexicon is continually evolving to the point where even members of the same generation that devised this term can't agree on its meaning. I asked several hundred undergraduate students to define the term you hear all the time, "hooking up." The range of responses was limitless, from going out for a cup of coffee, making out, anything but some form of penetration, to vaginal sex. My favorite response was the one I received from five different women who all defined hooking up as "random oral sex!"

In *Unhooked, Washington Post* journalist Laura Sessions Stepp's excellent commentary on contemporary sexual mores, she makes the point that using ambiguous terms like "hooking up" provides a person the freedom to do whatever he/she likes and not feel embarrassed or awkward afterward.

Quoting a college professor, Stepp suggests, for example, that it's easier for a young woman to say "I hooked up with a guy last night," than it would be to say "I gave this guy whose name I don't remember a blow job." I can now see its appeal.

I'd like some sex. Is simply asking someone out of the question?

An old college friend of mine we'll call Alan (because that was his name) subscribed to the crushingly honest but stunningly insensitive strategy of simply asking women if they'd like to have sex with him, pretty much as soon as he met them. All this was done face-to-face with barely a blush, and in Alan's estimation produced a positive result about 10 percent of the time, saving, in his opinion, time, effort, and considerable sums of money.

Today's technological highway of sexual seduction has, in a sense, mimicked my old pal's method. When a man texts a woman at midnight to ask if she wants to "hang out," he's probably asking Alan's question. The intentionally vague nature of "hanging out" allows for freedom of both expectation and deed and makes the asking of the question less threatening to both parties. Alan would have loved being in college today!

Is oral sex sex?

About a year before anyone had heard the name Monica Lewinsky and cigars were for smoking, a survey asked college students whether or not they believed oral sex and anal sex counted as *having* sex. The vast majority of respondents believed that neither counted as having sex. To which I reply: then what the heck are they? Whether or not this percep-tion has been spawned in reaction to the conserva-tive right's obsession with abstinence until marriage is unclear, but what is most worrisome is the implicit assumption by many that oral and anal sex are safe activities simply because pregnancy is not an issue. Despite the efforts of the abstinence-only advocates, unmarried men and women continue to have sex, and studies show that adolescents engage in oral sex more frequently than vaginal sex. Transmission of sexually transmitted infections are quite possible through both oral and anal sex and are discussed in gloriously graphic details in Part Three: The Other Stuff.

If I haven't had sex for a year, can I regain my virginity?

The answer to this one is definitely no. In these bizarre times where virginity is next to godliness, a number of adolescents, mainly female, are attempting to erase a forgettable night of awkward sex by promising to abstain from sex until they marry. Who's kidding who? If you've had sexual intercourse you can't be a virgin—again. Sorry. We could, of course, wait a year and see if your hymen grows back. And when it doesn't, the answer will still be a resounding no. Hav-ing said that, there's absolutely nothing wrong with waiting to have sex again if you feel like you're not ready or just don't want to do it. Despite what you might see and hear, having sex is *not* a mandatory activity.

Do men/women like virgins?

The majority of men I've asked this question respond, "It depends." If the man is really into the woman, then he's fine with it. However, if the evening is, say, "recreational," then most men say an emphatic "no," as they don't want the responsibility, or the potential "stage five clinger" aftermath, as one young man described. Men fear they'll get stalked if they're someone's "first." Interesting, almost without exception, heterosexual women seemingly have no use for virgins. They want men with a little experience. I once heard one young man say, "Thank God I had sex before I came to college!"

Why do some men have so much trouble taking enough direction on how to give a woman an orgasm?

Does the man care whether or not you have an orgasm? Just thought I'd throw that out for your consideration since we know that there are at least a couple of men around who care only about their own satisfaction. Having got that out of the way, how well have you provided the all-important directions? We all know how difficult it is to talk about sex. Some women might feel they're giving explicit directions when they're actually only hinting. Don't forget, some of us men need to be hit over the head with a large object to get our attention, so this is not the time to be subtle.

The other factor that should be considered here is that the woman's road to achieving an orgasm, in many cases, is much more circuitous and complicated than the male's. If the male's trip is 120 miles per hour down the fast lane of a straight highway, the woman's sojourn involves maps, satellite navigation, and several pit stops in uncharted locales, with no certain confidence that the end point will ever be reached. Don't give up on the teaching. Be absolutely explicit and definitive about what you like or need. He'll catch on eventually.

My boyfriend has an ex-girlfriend who calls him all the time. They sometimes meet for lunch, but he insists there's nothing going on—they're just good friends. What do you think?

I think he's having sex—or wants to! I subscribe to the When Harry Met Sally theory. If you haven't already, watch *When Harry Met Sally* and pay close attention to Billy Crystal's character, Harry, when he explains to Meg Ryan's character, Sally, that men can't be friends with women they find attractive. According to Harry, men will always have the opportunity for sex in the back of their minds, so no matter how much they might insist that they can be friends with someone, the possibility of sex is always looming. Increasing the likelihood of sex is Harry's admission when Sally suggests that men can only be friends with women they find unattractive. Harry replies, "No, you pretty much want to nail them too." No question, according to the majority of men, the When Harry Met Sally theory rules, so the odds say your boyfriend is doing her—or at least wants to.

I have a guy friend who stops by once or twice a week and we have sex, no strings attached. I'm beginning to have feelings for the guy—what's the chance we could have a relationship?

"Friends with benefits." The ideal relationship—great sex, longer lived than a one-night stand, and no commitment or hang-ups. Too good to be true? A recent study performed at Michigan State University that surveyed college students suggested that around 60 percent of the students sampled reported having had at least one "friend with benefits," with the most common reason being not wanting commitment. In only 10 percent of the cases did the friendship develop into a relationship, about 30 percent ended the sex but stayed friends, around 25 percent stopped both the sex and the friendship, and the remainder kept on sharing the benefits. So, according to these statistics, the chances of your friendship morphing into a committed relationship are pretty slim, but you won't know if you don't try. Talk to him.

Is there an easy way to ask someone how many partners they've had?

Hey, some people would be only too thrilled to tell you they've boffed dozens of partners, and others would certainly be willing to exaggerate—or understate—their résumé. The important issue is *why* you're asking the question in the first place. If it's to determine whether or not your new partner has had sex with half the state, if he's a man, you can, for the most part, make that assumption. But if you're trying to determine your relative risk for some sexually transmitted infection, although there is a relationship between the number of partners your new friend has had and the likelihood that he or she may have an infection, your question does not guarantee you'll get some accurate or helpful information. A more effective question might be, "Do you always use condoms when you have sex?" Think about it. A person who uses a condom 100 percent of the time with thirty partners might be a safer sexual risk than someone who has had as few as three partners but only occasionally used condoms.

What's the average number of sexual partners for men and women?

That's an interesting question, because most people tend to overestimate the average number. One of the most well-designed and representative studies of

American sexual behavior since Kinsey was published in 1994. This study, *Sex in America,* suggested that the average number of sexual partners in a lifetime is six for men and two for women. These numbers seem amazingly conservative and make me wonder if any of the study subjects ever went to college! Do numbers really matter? Probably not, except when some men see their own numbers lagging behind the average, they might feel the need for a rapid increase to keep up with the quota. A more recent survey of a representative sample of Americans aged 21–49 reported much higher numbers with an average of fourteen for men and eleven for women. These numbers seem a bit more realistic.

Why do some men insist on pushing your head down onto their crotch when you're making out? Couldn't they be more subtle?

I have now officially heard this complaint a thousand times! A man and woman are having a good time fooling around, when suddenly the woman feels a strange pressure on the back of her head that seems to be pushing her downward toward the man's crotch. Thinking that all those watermelon shooters have made her head feel heavy, the woman tries to raise her torso, but to no avail. The constant pressure on the back of her head is equaled only by a vague impression that the man's crotch is actually moving upward like a silent elevator. The collision is inevitable.

What a lot of women don't understand is that this motion is the male's "subtle" way of asking for oral sex. "Will you go down on me?" or "Will you suck my dick?" is clearly too blunt. The average man knows full well that being so direct would be in poor taste. Hence—in his mind at least—this unspoken communication is both subtle and directional.

Let's be honest, men have been doing the same with their partners' hands since forever. They're having a great time, lots of great foreplay, passionate kissing, and suddenly the guy takes her hand in his. "Oh," she thinks, "he's going to look deep into my eyes and tell me how much I mean to him." Then she notices that for some reason his hand is drawing her hand downward, lower and lower, until finally his palm pushes her hand against his erection and the implied request is all too obvious.

Personally, I'd suggest a little role reversal. Grab the guy by his hair, jam his head firmly between your legs, and tell him to take care of business down there before he starts pushing *your* head down. He might just get the message. Of course, a more constructive alternative might be to actually communicate and talk about what it is you want—or don't want.

How do I persuade my girlfriend to agree to a threesome? What should I tell her?

Tell her the third person's going to be a guy—that might be more persuasive! What's the matter? Lost your enthusiasm all of a sudden? Funny how men nearly always assume that the ménage à trois will be with an extra woman. Surely if you want to double your pleasure with another woman in the bed, wouldn't fairness dictate that you offer the same opportunity to your woman? What's that you say? It's *different*? Oh, right, I'd forgotten that all females are essentially bisexual and are just waiting for the opportunity to sample another woman for *both* your sakes.

I'm not sure that "persuade" is the right way to go. Broach the subject every now and again and if she's up for it, I'm sure she'll let you know. But do be prepared for her to voice her equal right to have an additional penis in the bed. It's only fair.

How can I talk about improving my girlfriend's sexual technique without hurting her feelings?

In the world of leadership and personnel management, one of the prevailing principles is to compliment someone first and then constructively criticize. So a conversation could go like this, "When you give me head, your lips feel so soft and wonderful, but your teeth feel like they're stripping a goddamn ear of corn, so please take it easy."

I don't think your girlfriend will be sucking anything but air after that statement, so try including the compliment and then following it not by a direct criticism but a constructive suggestion. "When you give me head, your lips feel so soft and wonderful, and I *really* like it when you . . ." (You can be thinking "keep your teeth to yourself" but don't say it, just fill in the blank with a sweeter suggestion.)

What exactly is date rape and how common is it?

The term "date or acquaintance rape" was pretty much coined in the 1980s. Does that mean date rape didn't happen prior to that date? No, many men just called it seduction or foreplay. The general public became aware through high-profile cases like that of the boxer Mike Tyson, who was convicted in 1992 of raping Miss Black Rhode Island, Desiree Washington, in an Indianapolis hotel and Kobe Bryant's brush with the law for sexual assault in 2003, though charges against him were dropped. Cases receiving zero publicity happen all the time, and I would certainly consider date rape as a major problem on most if not all college campuses, although because of the lack of formal reporting, exact numbers are impossible to obtain.

Date rape is when two people who know each other get together and some form of penetration occurs that is unwanted by one of the partners. The vast majority of date rape occurs between men and women but other combinations, like male on male, female on female, and even female on male are possible. I honestly believe that most people don't understand what date rape "looks like." Forget the exaggerated stereotype of the male physically beating a female into submission and then savagely raping her. I'm not saying that never happens—of course it does—but it's not the typical scenario. Much more likely is when two people are attracted to each other so they hook up (usually wasted to the point of stupor), and sex occurs. From what he remembers, he thinks they've had a great night. She, on the other hand, believes she's been raped. What a mess.

The gold standard of date-rape definitions seems to be that there must be verbal consent, in this example, by the female. Obviously, if both partners are wasted, verbal consent is unlikely to be asked for or given, so most laws simplify that problem and suggest that if the woman is so drunk as to be unable to provide consent, than subsequent intercourse will be considered rape.

Alcohol plays a *huge* role in date rape cases, along with our total inability to communicate meaningfully about sex. Think about it. In sexual situations, how much conversation or verbal communication actually occurs? Most sexual activity involves a lot of sweaty groping, panting, gasping, hands placed here and there, removed from here and there, and so on. Research shows that the majority of penis-vagina intercourse with a new partner involves zero discussion, which is possibly fine if the sex is absolutely consensual on both sides. The gray area is where one partner (stereotypically the woman) is less certain that she wants to have sex. She may already have had oral sex but, of course, that's just a contemporary handshake, so what does that really mean? It's understandably difficult for anyone who's just had his penis worked over to gasp out, "You've just performed amazing oral sex, does that mean we can follow up with a vigorous bout of penis-vagina intercourse?" Who's able to choke that out? Sprinkle large amounts of alcohol over this situation and meaningful communication becomes almost impossible.

The crucial point here is, if the guy is doubtful for one millisecond that his partner is hesitant about having sex, he better damn well ask the question before it's too late. Many guys don't want to ask as it does afford the woman an opportunity to come to her senses and decline sex, leaving the male cursing his thoughtfulness. Better that, though, than the potential tragedy that can follow unwanted sex.

Are men generally the ones who end relationships?

Actually, some social psychology research has suggested that women tend to dump men more than vice versa, but you have to be careful interpreting statistics. Ending a relationship face-to-face is one conflict the male of the species will avoid because they know that what follows is a lengthy and complex analysis led by the female of what went wrong and what could possibly be done to salvage things.

This is anathema to a man, as he's already put the issue behind him—it's in the vault, done, over, and all he wants to do is move on. And so the male antidote to his predicament was created.

The male simply treats his partner like absolute crap for several weeks, or even months (he can be so patient when need be), until finally she's had enough and tells him that if this is how things are going to be, then it's over. Feigning disappointment (but not too much, lest she feel sad and reconsider), he reluctantly agrees that they should break up.

Along comes the social psychologist to survey who dumped whom, and of course, the check goes in the female column. Like I said, interpreting statistics can be tricky.

I have a history of cheating on my boyfriends. Should I tell my new partner about my past?

In a perfect world, total honesty about ourselves might be the ultimate gold standard of communication. In the real world, if you tell your new partner about your history of consistent infidelity, I'm thinking that chances are you'll have no new relationship to worry about! Unless your boyfriend has an ego the size of Rhode Island, I can't imagine him embracing the idea that somehow you'll be different this time. Every time you're late meeting him, his mind will morph to a visual of you enjoying meaningless but dynamite sex with the checkout guy from the local supermarket. How productive is that? What's past is past—all you can control are your present actions. But if you do fall off the monogamy train and land squarely on a penis, *then* you need to start talking to your partner about your little problem.

Dumping by phone . . . fax . . . texting . . . IM . . . what's the protocol?

Dumping someone by phone was once thought to be pretty tacky. Today, you can dump someone by text message as you drive to work, or perhaps IM him or her as you download some new music. Although recent surveys suggest that only about 10 percent of Americans think that breaking up with a boyfriend or girlfriend by text message is OK, that percentage will inevitably increase as technology continues to dominate our lives.

Here are a few examples of how that's already happening today. For a small price one service called The Breakup Butler will attach a voice message to an e-mail that painlessly (at least for the person who hired the service) terminates a relationship. Goodbye Bitch is a Web site that provides a message generator to help rid you of an unwanted mate, while another service provides a prerecorded telephone voice-mail line that will tell someone who was given the number that a would-be lover isn't interested in him or her.

Finally, the pièce de résistance is the automated

e-mail message you can order anonymously to tell someone that he or she may have been infected with a sexually transmitted infection and should get checked out. Now that's communication! Ultimately, the right thing to do in a committed relationship gone bad is to talk face-to-face, but the temptation of using technology will be just too great for many people.

Has technology influenced the way we communicate about sex?

It has, and in so many ways. Just think about how difficult many people found using the telephone to ask someone out. Dial four digits, hang up. Dial five digits, then hang up again. Finally get through and stammer out some pathetic request that is greeted by the most dreaded phone response in recorded history, "Who is this, again?"

It's so much easier to write things in a message and send it off into the ether—no stumbling, no fumbling, just words that you could have rehearsed and crafted for hours. Admittedly, reading between the lines by picking up on voice inflections is missing from electronic communication, but you were usually so freaked out on the phone you couldn't hear the inferences anyway.

The ease of electronic communication does come at a potential cost. Because you're not physically talking to a person, there may be a tendency to be more flirtatious, bold, or risqué in your messaging that sends an exciting but perhaps misleading subtext to the receiver. (Regard texting and IM-ing as the equivalent of three-drink conversation and you'll get the idea.) Then when you actually get together in the flesh, so to speak, the assumptions that have been made from your electronic communication provide a difficult and sometimes even misleading reality. Maybe stammering on the phone has its uses!

Do people seriously hook up with other people they meet online?

Despite all the lurid tales of individuals hooking up with someone they met online only to disappear and be discovered six months later in separate garbage bags in a local landfill, it seems that, for some, the temptation is too great to resist. According to a survey performed by the Beta Research Corporation in 2006, 14 percent of men and 11 percent of women met their current sexual partners online. Maybe the risk is part of the rush? To be fair, more and more individuals are meeting online, and as long as they remember to take precautions like meeting in a public place and not going home together (yet), the Internet can be a positive date-generating technology. Beware also of online profiles, where typically women tend to understate weight and age, while men can be less than candid about their height, income, age, and marital status.

Although I have a girlfriend, I've been flirting by text message with another woman. Does this count as cheating?

This is a perfect example of technological advances outstripping traditionally defined sexual mores. Back in the day, having sex with another person, writing sexually explicit letters, or making dirty phone calls would be universally accepted as cheating. But what do we do with all this messaging stuff? President Carter, in an interview with *Playboy* magazine in 1976 while governor of Georgia, admitted lusting after other women and therefore committing adultery in his heart. I guess only the person doing the texting knows what's really going on. Odds are, though, that (even electronic) flirting will lead to some sort of physical behavior, so let's err on the side of safety here. If you're flirting with your keypad, you're probably cheating, at least in your heart.

Is there any difference between the sexes when it comes to text messaging?

Recent research confirms that although men primarily use messaging as a tool for managing their relationships, women often view text as an additional means to develop an emotional connection. Although both sexes will use messaging to make arrangements, change plans, confirm times, make dates, and even end relationships, men are a lot more likely to do so. Let's face it, messaging is an absolute godsend to a sex that hates uncomfortable, emotional interactions, where even a phone call is fraught with breathy silences and unavoidable angst. Messaging avoids that uncomfortable connection and because of its format, gets the point across in a direct manner, without a lengthy and emotional explanation.

Although texting provides near-instant gratification, Simeon Yates of Sheffield Hallam University in England, lead researcher of a technology study in conjunction with Virgin Media, observes that messaging isn't always a positive concept; "It's a way for some daters to do less, act as if they care less and, in doing so, gain the upper hand in a relationship," he says. Texting may indeed afford the opportunity for instant communication, but clearly the subtext is not always a positive one.

Yates also tracked the average length of text messages—men messaging women, seventy words; women messaging men, eighty words; women messaging women, eighty-five words; and men messaging men, six words. Men clearly don't want to waste any time communicating with each other.

Does messaging help men avoid rejection?

Of course. Again, eons ago, before the world of electronics, many men would approach women face-to-face or by telephone and experience the stinging lash of rejection with all the accompanying feelings of emasculation. Text messaging allows the suitor to flirt and gauge interest levels without embarrassment, and if the recipient isn't interested, there's simply no reply. It's all very painless, and much less threatening to the all too fragile masculine ego.

A guy I'm seeing basically refuses to talk to me on the phone. When I call him he constantly makes excuses to hang up, then texts me immediately afterward and tries to have a conversation. Is this typical, because it's really annoying me!

I'm not sure how common this is, but your situation certainly confirms the idea that texting has been embraced by many people, both men and women, who seem to prefer this less personalized and more facile method of communication. I find it hard to conceive of how your friend is able to handle face-to-face conversation. Some individuals hate to talk on the phone, so perhaps that might have something to do with his reticence, but I'd suggest asking him (to his face) why he has such a problem talking on the phone, and see where that takes you. There's a clear need here to communicate.

Call the morning after? Or text?

My suggestion would be that if you're truly interested in pursuing a relationship, pick up the phone. Failing that, perhaps send a brief but endearing text message to the effect that you had a great time last night. I don't believe that social mores have established a minimum-time-before-you-text-someone protocol, so don't get into playing those mind games; get in touch. I think what you say is more important than which medium you use to say it.

Should I turn off my cell phone during sex?

A recent study found that only one in seven British respondents turned off their cell phones before having sex. Are we so desperate to be available and in touch with the world that we have to leave our phones on during sex? I guess the real acid test would be how many people actually respond to a call during their episode of passion. Never too busy to take a call? Unless you're using the vibration mode for mind-blowing purposes, I think etiquette (and any hopes of great sex) would dictate that you turn off your phone, for just a few minutes anyway.

PART TWO:

Everything You Really Should Know About Sex

Before Sex, During Sex, and After Sex

What makes us respond to various sexual stimuli? What makes our pulse race, our skin flush, our head swim with sexual tension? What factors exist that influence how we react to different messages and signals around us? While no one can say for sure, researchers have identified some important factors that seem to have varying degrees of influence on our sexual response. Genetics and hormones play a large role in this process for animals lower down the evolutionary chain, but because humans are so "big brained," this large organ between our ears is the most important influence on our reaction to sexual stimuli. Many experts in the field believe that a large proportion of our responses are basically learned through the powerful effects of socialization.

If we examine stereotypical sexual turn-ons in our culture, it would be difficult to argue that women are genetically programmed to feel sexy when wearing Chanel No.5 perfume or wearing leather miniskirts. The sex appeal associated with clothing is purely temporal—fashions come and go—and culture specific. If you doubt me, get one of your parents to pull out some photos that date back to their youth. The clothes that seemed so hip and sexy back then will be ridiculed by contemporary fashion mavens as old, unfashionable, and tawdry. The only consolation that we mature folks have is that the arrogant youth of today will in turn be put on the rack by their own children, victims of each new generation's need to redefine itself as condescendingly superior.

Before Sex

Is there a time in the menstrual cycle when women are more receptive to having sex?

If the answer to this question was a clear-cut yes, it could certainly streamline and maximize the efforts taken to have sex. Female dogs, for example, experience a surge of estrogen called "estrus" about four times a year, signaling that they are "in heat" to male dogs in the vicinity. I've often thought the male-female mating ritual would be greatly simplified if a man could enter a bar, sniff, and say, "I smell estrus, come on, who's ready?" Just a thought, but it would certainly save time and several drinks.

Human females don't work this way. Theoretically, a woman should *want* to have intercourse most when she is ovulating (see next question) so that she's more likely to get pregnant (that's why your body is having sex!). However, research has shown that although some women might report individual preferences, there is no overall consensus as to when a woman is most interested in sex. It's an individual thing, and again, it's because of that big-brain influence.

When do women ovulate and why should we care?

Most men—and a high proportion of women—sadly can't answer this question. First, for the information challenged, a simple definition of ovulation is: the time when a woman's body produces an ova or egg that is viable and able to be fertilized. This is great information to have as it could actually help you get pregnant when you finally want to, or alternately, a heterosexual couple might have philosophical or religious beliefs that preclude them from using contraception, so knowing a little bit about menstrual cycles could help them make an informed decision. (Being too lazy, drunk, or just plain out of it are not good-enough reasons to use this knowledge about ovulation as a form of contraception.) A woman usually ovulates fourteen days *before* her next menstrual period, not *after* her last one. The idea here is that because sperm can live for approximately seventy-two hours once they enter the vagina, cervix, uterus, and fallopian tubes, if you can work out when a woman ovulates and then avoid intercourse about three days before and after that day, you could reduce the likelihood of pregnancy.

The problem is that Mother Nature is essentially a tease. If all women ovulated fourteen days *after* their last period, this method would be foolproof. Anyone smart enough to count to fourteen would be able to use it. But instead, Mother Nature makes it fourteen days *before* her next period, a much less predictable time. Many women also have unpredictable cycles in general, which means you'll have as much luck with forecasting ovulation as you will with the weather.

According to advocates of this method (also known as the rhythm method, or natural family planning), effectiveness rates for preventing pregnancy range from 99 percent to a much more conservative 75 percent from other sexual-health professionals. If you're really motivated to use this method, you can do some research on "natural family planning" or "fertility" but you're going to need to be very motivated.

Negotiating sex: as a guy, do I need my lawyer?

If you're even asking that question, the answer is probably yes. Because of all the high-profile publicity about sexual assault and date rape, men in particular have become a little more aware about the potential pitfalls of any activities remotely associated with sex. I'm not sure you need a lawyer, but what you *don't* need to do is get so drunk that you have no idea what's going on, can't hear what's being said by your potentially less than enthusiastic partner, and ultimately only be able to tell the judge that sex did take place, but you can't remember anything else.

Two important things for every man to consider (that will help you to avoid needing a lawyer):

- don't get so wasted that you don't know what you're doing, or what your partner might be trying to tell you
- if you are in *any* doubt about what your partner wants, ASK!

Are oysters really aphrodisiacs?

An aphrodisiac is something that will increase your libido or sex drive, and legend seems to have it that oysters are just the crustaceans to do the job, to the point where a man can't order a dozen oysters in a restaurant without the waiter giving him a sideways look. As with other supposed aphrodisiacs like ginseng, chocolate (including green M&Ms!), and Spanish fly, there is usually a tiny grain of possible truth to the notion, although never enough to make a legitimate claim. Oysters are rich in zinc, a mineral assumed to be a sexual response enhancer, but that's a far cry from being a substance that has been documented as increasing libido.

What's a true aphrodisiac?

The only known true aphrodisiac is . . . wait for it . . . variety. Think about it! Seriously though, there's no substance that is proven to actually increase your libido. However, the good news is that many experts believe a placebo effect can occur. That is, if you believe something will increase your sex drive, you might feel more aroused, and that's great for you, but your perceived state has nothing to do with the supposed aphrodisiac.

Alcohol has to be an aphrodisiac, right?

Alcohol seems like it should be an aphrodisiac. It can make you feel great, but actually, it can't possibly be a sexual stimulant, because chemically it's a central nervous system depressant. Ask any man the effects of alcohol when he's had one drink too many. He goes from a god who just knows he can last all night to a nothing who will have to roll over and sleep off his embarrassment. Rather than being an aphrodisiac, alcohol is actually an inhibition relaxer. It's an automatic excuse for a man when he sleeps with a socially unacceptable partner. "Dude, I was wasted, I didn't know what the hell I was doing!" It's an automatic excuse for a woman when she doesn't want to appear too easy, or she's had sex with someone perceived as less than acceptable. "I don't know how that happened. I was so, like, toasted."

I hear that Viagra increases your sex drive. Is that true?

Only in your dreams—literally! If you take Viagra and you *think* it increases your libido and sex is much better, then congratulations, but your response had nothing to do with the drug. Viagra does not increase your sex drive. Viagra is intended for use by men experiencing problems with erectile dysfunction and is not intended for improving the romping, recreational sex of twentysomethings! Unfortunately, it only takes one moron to get on the Internet and brag about how Viagra gave him the boner of all boners and how he went at it all night long before every guy around the world is slapping down his ten dollars for a piece of that action. Viagra could prove to be less than the bargain you hoped for if you're one of the men who dies from a Viagra-induced heart attack. Just a thought.

Why can't men understand that foreplay is just as, if not more, important than sex itself?

For most heterosexual men, sex is a fairly linear experience. It begins with kissing (if you're lucky), moves to fondling, possibly to oral sex and mutual masturbation, then concludes with penis-vagina intercourse and hopefully, not too soon, an all-too-brief orgasm. The reason for rushing the hors d'oeuvres and stampeding toward the main course may be related to the fact that most men have spent their youth masturbating themselves silly, fantasizing what having sex with a real, warm, breathing person might feel like. So although having that other person's hand around might make for a nice change, the real thrill, the total buzz, is undoubtedly sexual intercourse.

I also think at the back of many men's minds is the paranoia that having sex is simply too good to be true. He'd better get inside her before she changes her mind or her parents come home or her roommate kicks him out or some other frustrating scenario from a bad movie happens. Oh, the pressure!

Another factor that cannot be ignored is, again, the male may not understand or even care about the female's need for more prolonged foreplay, and will certainly never be able to relate to the idea that some women may not always orgasm during intercourse, but gain the most pleasure from prepenetrative sex. This clearly speaks to the importance and need for better communication between partners—you'd have no problem talking about the styles of food you like or your favorite movies or books. Being more open about our sexual likes and dislikes would certainly improve the chances for a more satisfying love life for both men and women.

How effective are condoms at preventing sexually transmitted infections?

Before I begin answering this question, here's the government-approved answer that you'll hear in a publicly funded sex education class: "Condoms are not 100 percent effective at preventing STIs. The only sure way to prevent an STI is total abstinence, and that includes no oral or anal sex."

Now that I've got that out of the way, let's provide some useful information. Here's an analogy. Can anyone guarantee that wearing a seat belt prevents you from being killed in an automobile accident? Of course not, but various studies estimate that seat belts are likely to be around 65 percent effective at reducing the likelihood of your death. So should we abandon wearing a device that could save our lives because of the failure rate? That wouldn't make much sense. Neither would refusing to use condoms just because they aren't 100 percent effective. Critics may question whether or not safe sex exists, but there is such a thing as safer sex.

Although some condoms are defective (an estimated fewer than 2 percent), "user" failure accounts for the vast majority of condom failure. You can't blame the condom and say it's ineffective if the user can't operate it correctly. I'm reminded of the scene in the movie *The 40-Year-Old Virgin* as the virgin hopelessly attempts to persuade several of his uncooperative latex friends to position themselves on his awaiting penis. The floor is littered with discarded condoms and appears as if rampant sex has occurred.

Here's the deal: when used correctly, latex condoms are around 98 percent effective at preventing most STIs, with prevention against human papilloma virus (genital warts) probably being a little less because of the possibility of warts on the base of the penis which the condom might not completely cover. The bottom line here is a simple one. If you're not prepared to be abstinent, then the only game in town to greatly reduce your risk for an STI is a latex condom, and if used correctly, the condom is around 98 percent effective. So use one!

When I put on a condom it feels really tight and I lose my erection. What's going on?

D
R

R
O
B
I
N

S
A
W
Y
E
R

What's going on with you is no doubt embarrassing and a real pain, but it's actually not uncommon. Let's start with a positive. The condom may be too tight because you have an enormous penis. There, feeling better? You could try a more accommodating condom like the Trojan Magnum or LifeStyles King Size XL. There is a set of condoms specially designed for men who feel like the head of their penis is being suffocated, and they are manufactured with a flared bulb-like head to create more space. Examples include Elexa Natural Feel or Trojan Her Pleasure condoms. If you're still having problems after the larger condom, then I recommend that you consult a sex therapist as the problem may not be physical.

Men should also be aware that the opposite problem, wearing a condom that is too loose, increases risk for both STIs and unintended pregnancy. The reality is that most men don't like wearing condoms, but they do need to pay greater attention to the issue of fit. A recent study performed by the condom manufacturer Durex reported that 50 percent of condom users felt that the condoms they regularly used didn't fit properly, 25 percent said condoms were too tight, 10 percent said much too tight, and 15 percent said too loose. The condom industry is currently lobbying for a greater range in sizes on the very reasonable assertion that no other body parts come in a uniform size. Some experts believe that if condoms fit better and felt more comfortable, men might be more willing to use them consistently.

If the condom slips, particularly during or after sex, it's too loose. Few companies have offered smaller sizes, so if slippage is an issue, try a different brand that might work better for you. If the condom feels like it's pinching the penis to the point of discomfort, chances are you need a bigger size. Check out some of the examples listed above.

How do you ask someone if they've had an HIV test?

A better question to ask yourself might be, does asking someone if they've had an HIV test really serve a useful purpose? Despite all the politically correct propaganda to the contrary, asking someone if he or she has had an HIV test is still akin—in many people's minds—to asking if they're some kind of sleaze who's shagged half the population and who's probably incubating an indescribably foul disease as we speak. The real question is, do you want to put yourself and the other person through all this mental angst if the answer you can obtain has no real value?

The result of a person's HIV test is only useful the day he or she receives it. At that point, HIV status is unequivocally known, but days and weeks after that point, the result has less value, if any. Unless you and your partner both have an HIV test at exactly the same time, knowing that someone was tested six months ago tells you nothing useful because anything could have happened since that time. If you and a new partner get to the point where intercourse is imminent, the best way to handle this type of request is to suggest you both go for testing together. You'll be company for each other and know exactly where you stand with HIV.

After about twenty minutes of performing oral sex on my partner, my jaw starts to ache and I can't feel my face . . . what should I do?

This begs the oral-sex protocol question: "How long is reasonable?" Let's think: chronic jaw ache, totally numb face, and you've been working on that thing for twenty minutes? Come on, it's way past time to move on. Some people will want a shorter session so they can get to the Holy Grail, the intercourse, while others may view oral sex as the end point. Even so, if you've been working diligently on that thing to the extent that you don't even know what you're sucking anymore, it's time to call it quits. The recipient is just lying back, taking advantage. They need to get their head in the game, and move on. The $60,000 question is would they be down between your legs for an eon, getting lockjaw? Maybe, but maybe not. The reality is that although oral sex may be great for the recipient, extended head time can be very tiring and uncomfortable for the donor. I say, unless both partners are comfortable with marathon sessions, let's put a time limit on the business—some point before the face becomes stricken with paralysis!

How do I transition out of oral sex with my boyfriend without making it obvious that I don't like it?

First, here's what not to do. Don't hold the penis between your forefinger and thumb as if it's some offensive dog turd; don't make a face like you just smelled something bad; don't dry heave, as that tends to ruin the moment; and don't mutter, "God, this is gross" as his penis leaves your mouth. What you *can* do to transition is whisper, "I can't wait to feel you inside me" while throwing your leg over him, rolling on a condom, and inserting the penis before he has a chance to complain that the oral stimulation only lasted ten seconds.

Of course, the other alternative—crazy as it might sound—is to talk to your partner about not being that comfortable with oral sex. The longer anyone does something sexually they don't really like or enjoy, the faster resentment will build and problems will inevitably follow. Talk about it.

Could having sex before an important game hurt my athletic performance?

This question has been debated for years, and given the amount of money in collegiate and professional sports, you can see why it might be important. The consensus of the research tends to suggest that although you probably shouldn't be up all night having hot sex the night before the Olympic 100-meter final, adhering to your regular pattern of sexual behavior leading up to the athletic event might not be a bad thing. Some research suggests that you might perform better feeling more relaxed since that can lead to less fatigue and more aerobic potential during the event.

Having said that, if you examine the philosophy of the leading teams in the World Cup, the world's largest sporting event, you might think differently. Italy has always been a team known for keeping girlfriends and wives away from players during competition, while England has been more relaxed about these issues. Italy has won the World Cup four times, the last occasion being in 2006. England has won the World Cup once, in 1966! Need I say more?

Why do guys like to watch porn so much?

To paraphrase a male student's response to this question in my class, "How can anyone *not* like porn? It's awesome!" Pornography, once the domain of seedy movie theaters in a bad part of town, has become almost mainstream these days, and young men in particular seem to appreciate this shift in social perception. Watching attractive people having sex can be extremely arousing for both men and women. In fact, erotica is often used during sexual therapy treatment to increase sexual arousal in individuals with low response levels. Men are very visually oriented and certainly for many, the next best thing to having sex is watching someone else do the deed. Of course, an interesting facet of erotica is the very brief amount of time actually spent watching the material, probably about five minutes in most cases.

My boyfriend and I watch X-rated movies a lot when we have sex, and we both get really turned on. I'm just getting a little worried because we never seem to have sex without watching the movies. Do you think it's a problem?

I think it's fair to say that for most men, there's probably no such thing as too much porn. Men's capacity to consume erotica is only surpassed by their ability to masturbate anytime, anywhere. However, there is a genuine concern that some men are becoming addicted to porn, particularly on the Internet. In a heterosexual relationship, a man's insistence on watching porn every time before sex is certainly likely to be interpreted by his female partner to mean that she's somehow inadequate and that the man can't respond without the added erotic boost. In most cases, that probably isn't true and the man is at worst a little lazy and at best just enjoys the buzz he gets from erotica. Maybe suggest that you have sex without the "professional assistance," perhaps substituting the celluloid sex for something more romantic. Obviously if your man won't or can't perform without his usual fix of porn, then potentially you do have a more serious problem and need to seek help.

Contraception: Pregnancy
Is Avoidable

Since the dawn of civilization, women have been trying to prevent pregnancy. We've come a long way since biblical times, when women combined crocodile dung and honey in a desperate attempt to plug the cervix. And although Victorian women progressed to a more gastronomically pleasant-sounding concoction called contraceptive fudge, effectiveness was little better.

Although contraception might seem to be a straight-forward issue to most people today, some individuals consider it to be controversial, often because of religious beliefs. The notion that birth control interferes with the natural process of becoming pregnant is a problem for people who feel that contraception should not be used because it is interfering with God's will. Until relatively recently, states had laws making contraception illegal, and even today we continue to see individual pharmacists refusing to fill prescriptions for contraception because it is against their religious beliefs. How weird is that? Ever heard of a job description?

I wonder if these pharmacists also refuse to fill prescriptions for Viagra on the basis that gerontological intercourse (I suppose that's anyone over forty according to anyone under thirty) is pretty unlikely to result in pregnancy and therefore goes against the religious belief that sex is only for procreation? In a culture where only a limited number of insurance companies cover the cost of women's contraception but nearly all cover a man's expenses for Viagra, you have to ask yourself, What's it all about? Insurance companies aren't willing to pay for the costs of female contraception because sex clearly isn't absolutely necessary for women, but we have to subsidize the guy who needs help getting a boner? Oh well, who said sex made sense?

We've come a long way since the times when the only available contraceptive method was a condom. Although the list isn't long, we are now able to choose from a variety of methods that if used correctly can effectively prevent pregnancy. Hopefully this section will help you with making that choice. Before I get to answering your "During Sex" questions, I want to address—in full—contraception, which is something I hope *you* consider in full before deciding to have sex.

The perfect method of contraception?

Let's be fair, no method of contraception exists that anyone actually likes to use. So if you want to be an instant billionaire, in a world where contraception is a multimillion-dollar global business, design the perfect method of birth control. What features would earn it the title of "Perfecto"?

- 100 percent effectiveness against pregnancy
- 100 percent effectiveness against the transmission of STIs, including HIV
- Easy to use—nothing to strap on or lube up
- No interruption of foreplay
- Either sex could use the method
- Perfecto works instantly so you don't have to use a backup method
- No negative side effects—in fact, this method makes you feel damn good!
- Perfecto increases the likelihood of orgasm in women (see "why the hell can't I orgasm?" in the Dysfunction section).
- Perfecto is instantly reversible, meaning as soon as a couple ends use, the woman can get pregnant
- To encourage use, the method is federally funded and free

So, Perfecto's looking pretty good? Who wouldn't want these attributes in a method of contraception? Although it's fun to fantasize, the cruel reality is that you'll never see Perfecto on the market. All we have to choose from is a group of methods that have some of these features. But before we have a pity party, at least these methods are available and you do have some choices. A couple of generations ago all that existed were some condoms and a lot of prayer, not the most effective of methods. Although today's list is indeed limited, and all the methods have some flaws, you're able to select the best of the bunch for you and your situation.

So how do I go about selecting a method?

Here are some questions to ask yourself that might help:

- *Am I forgetful?* Be honest, are you a bit scatterbrained? If you are, using a method where you have to do something regularly, like taking the pill at the same time every day, might not be for you. Also, if you head to the mountains for a weekend of rampant sex and your condoms or diaphragm are back in town, you've got a dilemma!
- *Do I have any family or personal health problems that might rule out using a particular method?* Physicians estimate that about 10 percent of individuals can't use the more effective hormonal methods of contraception because of a personal or family history of health problems, such as cancer, stroke, migraines, etc.
- *Does interrupting sexual activity bother me?* Of

course being interrupted would bother anyone, but I guess the real question is, how much does it bother *you*? For example, if every time you have sex you have to stop to put on a condom, and that bugs you so much that sometimes you can't be bothered, then that method isn't for you.

- *Does having to remember to use something every time you have sex bother you?* Obviously, the advantage of the hormonal methods, unlike the condom, sponge, or diaphragm, is that you don't have to actually do anything to protect yourself against pregnancy every time you have sex. Some people don't mind that much, others hate having to remember.

- *How often do I have sex?* Examples: I'm a student at the University of Maryland and my boyfriend goes to college in California—we have sex about twenty times a year, should we just use condoms? My boyfriend and I both attend the University of Maryland and have sex about a thousand times a year, should we use oral contraception? The argument against taking hormones every day for limited amounts of sex is rational, but the bottom line is this: *the best method of contraception for you is the one you will actually use, correctly and consistently, regardless of frequency of intercourse.* If you hate a method, you won't use it consistently and are more likely to have a problem. Of course, for many individuals living in the less than monogamous community, condom use is essential to prevent STIs regardless of contraceptive choice.

- *Are you willing to put up with side effects?* Again, there's no free ride with contraception. For some women, the more effective hormonal methods can create some unpleasant side effects. For example, some women who use the pill may experience more yeast infections. Now, to the best of my knowledge, no woman has died from yeast infections, but a raging case of candidiasis isn't a lot of fun, so the woman is sometimes left with a difficult decision.

What's the most commonly used method of contraception for twenty and thirty-year-olds?

D
R

R
O
B
I
N

S
A
W
Y
E
R

The most common methods, and by "methods" I mean real, legitimate contraception, are oral contraception and condoms. I make that distinction because the other two "methods" I observe all too frequently on a college campus are prayer and withdrawal. The prayer is usually of a postintercourse type where the couple is so freaked out about the possible pregnancy that they've gone from atheists to acolytes before you can say holy wafer.

Needless to say, God doesn't always listen! Withdrawal, pulling out, or in my PhD vocabulary, *coitus interruptus*, is a very poor substitute for real contraception, mainly because a man's intention to withdraw is never quite matched by his ability to tug himself free before losing control, a sort of *coitus lostcontrollus*! There is also a theory that men's pre-ejaculatory fluid that is released prior to climax may contain live sperm from the last time the male ejaculated, meaning that even if a particular male keeps his cool, it may already be too late.

Do many people actually have sex without using contraception?

Anywhere from 30–50 percent of adolescents and younger adults fail to use contraception consistently. Scary, isn't it?! And although contraception use becomes more consistent with age, among women aged twenty-five and older, one-third to one-half of all pregnancies are unintended.

Why don't people use contraception?

That's an interesting question. I'm certainly not beating the prohibition drum, but my take on this is that if alcohol didn't exist, unintended pregnancy rates would be incredibly lower. Let's face it, many people are so freaked out about sex that they wouldn't even be doing it if it wasn't for alcohol. In the heterosexual world, it allows the man to pronounce the most ridiculous one-liners to women that he'd never say when sober, and permits the woman to think that the deliverer of the inane one-liner is cute, rather than the total asshole she'd consider him if she was sober. Also, there's the "beer goggle" or alcohol pseudo-aphrodisiac effect, enjoyed equally by both men and women.

Another major reason is the total denial that surrounds sex. In a study I performed on a college campus examining female students who had requested pregnancy tests, a large number of these women said they hadn't used contraception because they "hadn't expected sex to happen." Now come on, give me a break, this is total denial and rationalization. My definition of unexpected sex is when I've finished a lecture, a naked woman falls from the auditorium ceiling, and says, "Take me!" Now that would be unexpected!

Most young adults "hang out" for a while, maybe even make out a few times, and of course enjoy the splendors of a good session or two of oral sex, because today, that's just a means of getting to know someone. At some point, the couple will have done everything but penis-vagina sex, and then—can you believe it? They had sex!

Of course they had sex; I'd have bet my mortgage on it. Let me make an important point. For the most part, sex doesn't just happen. A young woman is not casually jogging down the street when she slips, flies through the air, does a somersault, and lands on a penis. This makes for a colorful visual image, but it's not real. We often don't plan for contraception because we'd rather not think about the implications of being sexually active, particularly on the female side of the street where society has punished women for exhibiting the same interest in sex as men.

A large number of people, particularly younger individuals, simply think "pregnancy won't happen to me." They may be well aware of all the facts and know intellectually that pregnancy could occur, but somehow the denial, and more often the alcohol, convinces them that this is someone else's problem.

When's the best time to talk with a partner about contraception?

The best time not to talk to a partner about the issue is at midnight, after a heavy bout of drinking, when you've been dry-humping for an hour, all clothes have been removed, and the penis is a millimeter from the vagina.

That's not a good time! The guy usually grunts out a dumb question like, "Are you on something?" The woman looks at him, trying to register what he's asking, thinking, "On something? What, like a freaking bicycle?" The woman isn't much better, though, as she gasps, "Do you have something?" He's buck naked, so his reply is "Well, not on me," as he freaks out wondering if the something she's referring to is a hidden case of genital warts!

As unromantic as it sounds, you need to take care of the contraceptive details long before you get to this point. Dealing with an unwanted pregnancy isn't very romantic either, to say nothing of a bad case of warts. The best time (and there's never really an easy or a best time) is when the possibility of intercourse is apparent to both of you. Talking about it may also have the added benefit of establishing that intercourse is actually going to occur and make both of you feel more relaxed about the whole thing.

I hate wearing condoms; is there anything else I could do instead?

Yeah, you could sit home and play with yourself. Quit whining. Sure, condoms aren't the greatest things in the world, but they're pretty effective at preventing pregnancy, and they're the only method of contraception that provides protection against those nasty sexually transmitted infections you want to avoid. The big knock on male condoms is that they reduce sensation, and that is a true statement. Condoms do reduce sensation and sometimes you might even wonder if you're actually having sex. But think of it this way, they also will reduce the likelihood of premature ejaculation. By the way, please don't put *two* condoms on in the vain hope that they'll double your hang time. This can cause tearing, so then you'll still end up embarrassed with the added bonus of a possible infection.

My boyfriend can't wear condoms, he bursts them. What can he do?

Who are you dating, Rambo? About 2–5 percent of condoms tear during use but most condom breakage occurs because the man doesn't use the condom correctly. Now, you don't have to be a rocket scientist to find your way around a condom but here are a few basics you and Rambo need to know.

- Don't get the penis anywhere near the vagina before putting on the condom, and if you're a guy, don't pull that pathetic, whiny, "Oh please, let me put it in for just a second before I put the condom on." Even if the guy has better staying power than a gnat, some experts believe that there's always an outside chance that his pre-ejaculatory fluid released prior to ejaculation may contain live sperm from the last ejaculation.

- If the condom feels way too loose or tight, you may need to find a different size or brand that will fit you better.

- To reduce the chance of your condom bursting or breaking, always make sure the condom's reservoir tip has sufficient space to be able to handle the semen. Hold the tip with your forefinger and thumb as you roll on the condom to make sure no air gets trapped, and do not used oil-based lubricants that could cause the condom to degrade and tear.

- Hold onto the condom as you withdraw the

penis after ejaculation. You don't want to leave it behind, and you should withdraw the penis soon after ejaculation as you'll lose a large proportion of your erection almost immediately after ejaculation.

- After holding up the condom to admire your studlike yield—come on, guys, you know you do that—dispose of the offending item responsibly and do not reuse!

How do you know if a condom is good before you use it?

The best indicator of a condom's condition is probably the expiration date on the outer wrapper. If your condom has passed its "sell by" or expiration date, you could well be using a defective rubber. So be sure your condom is still good according to the wrapper before you have your pants down. (By that point you'll probably have the lights out and can't see the expiration date, and quite frankly, if this is your first time, or first time in a long time, you won't give a damn if the date was 1867.)

Another practical tip: because the motor vehicle has become an oft-used location for a romantic tryst, many a condom has been placed in the glove compartment for storage. Given that the inside temperature of the car during the summer months in just about any U.S. state you'd care to mention is around 15,000 degrees, you can imagine what that heat will do to that poor little condom. Don't leave condoms in the car.

Are those condoms with spermicide better than the regular types at protecting against pregnancy or STIs?

Condoms with a spermicide coating (usually non-oxynol-9) are probably more effective than plain condoms at preventing STIs or pregnancy, but only very marginally. Although the vast majority of individuals use condoms with nothing else, the optimal way to use condoms is in conjunction with a spermicidal foam, cream, or gel. The spermicide is applied with a dispenser around the cervix and should probably be given about ten minutes to gain optimal protection before having intercourse. If you're using spermicide, you need to have intercourse within an hour—you can't go out for a quick drink before returning for postlibation sex, as your body temperature will melt the foam and it will run down your legs, obviously raising eyebrows at your local bar. To be honest, as a method of preventing pregnancy, I would consider a condom (assuming correct use) with an application of spermicidal foam almost as effective as the pill, with the obvious added advantage of STI prevention and much less risk of negative side effects.

Are female condoms any good?

Female condoms hit the American market in 1993, but you'll be glad if you didn't buy stock in the product. Made of polyurethane, the female condom has a smaller ring at the base of the condom, which is inserted into the vagina to cover the cervix, and a larger ring at the outer end that sits just outside the labia minora and prevents the condom from being pushed into the vagina. With movement during sex, the condom makes a definite rustling noise, so unless your "do me" music is turned up loud, it sounds like you're having sex with a shopping bag! Effectiveness rates at preventing pregnancy and/or STIs are vague, so this device on its own wouldn't be at the top of a hierarchy of effectiveness. If used in conjunction with the pill, the female condom provides extra protection. Overall, it's good that another option is available for women, but this condom is not considered as effective as its male counterpart at preventing pregnancy or STIs.

Is the sponge available again?

Any *Seinfeld* fan will remember Elaine's love of the contraceptive method called the sponge. Basically a one-size-fits-all diaphragm first introduced in 1983, the polyurethane sponge infused with a spermicide was taken off the market in 1995, and so the television episode showed Elaine hoarding the precious devices and having to make difficult decisions as to whether or not a man is worth the sacrifice of a sponge, or as she called it, "*sponge worthy*"!

In real life, after a ten-year hiatus, the sponge was returned to the marketplace, receiving FDA approval in 2005. A word of caution: used in conjunction with a condom it's a pretty good device, but the sponge on its own is as effective at preventing pregnancy as wrapping the penis in Saran Wrap. Let me ask you this, when have you ever worn something that was one-size-fits-all that actually fit? That would be never—you get my point?

Is Norplant still available?

No, Norplant's distribution in the United States ended in 2002. Norplant consisted of six rods implanted beneath the skin that released progestin, providing protection against pregnancy for up to five years. Norplant failed to win over sufficient numbers of adopters (particularly younger women) and there were also many complaints about the difficulty and discomfort involved in Norplant removal. Implanon, an extremely effective, single-rod device, received FDA approval in 2006 and is effective for up to three years.

Does Implanon have any side effects?

Side effects for Implanon are not dissimilar to those of oral contraception. Some women can experience one or more of the following: irregular or missed periods, break-through bleeding (spotting), weight gain, acne, headaches, breast tenderness, etc.

Is there a waiting period before oral contraception—the pill—takes effect?

If you're using a combination pill and take the initial pill within the first 5–6 days after the start of your period, the pill will be effective immediately. If you begin the pill outside that time frame, you'll need to use an additional form of contraception, like a condom, for at least the next seven days.

If you've been on the pill for five years, how long does it take for your body to become "regular" again?

Your body will return to its natural reproductive patterns and rhythms very quickly. Some practitioners advise waiting for a couple of menstrual cycles before trying to get pregnant, but there's really no data suggesting that getting pregnant the cycle after stopping the pill will be problematic.

If you're on the pill for several years, will it take longer to get pregnant after you stop taking it?

This is just another urban legend. Everyone's got a friend or relative with a story about the pill. "Aunt

Janet was on the pill for seven years and it took her eight more years to get pregnant after she stopped." Do we know how long it would have taken Janet to get pregnant had she never taken the pill?

Everyone tends to think they can get pregnant whenever they want, but sometimes life isn't that straightforward. Some women could have unprotected intercourse regularly for two years and not conceive while other women simply seem to look at a man and get pregnant. You know who you are! Nearly all young women have no idea about their fertility because they've been doing their best not to get pregnant. Most research would suggest that the pill has no effect on a woman's subsequent fertility.

Do you really have to take the pill at the same time every day?

When the pill was first introduced to the American marketplace in the 1960s, scientists wanted to ensure that ovulation didn't occur, so the levels of combined hormones were far in excess of what we find in today's lower-dose pills. However, the advantage that women of the sixties had was that they could probably forget to take the pill for several days and never get pregnant. Today's pills are considered to be much safer than the earliest version, but the downside is that they have a much smaller margin of error. To that end, women are advised, where possible, to take the pill at the same time every day.

I counseled a student one day who was pregnant and very angry because she was a meticulous pill taker—5:00 P.M. every day—and couldn't see how she'd gotten pregnant. We traced back the time of risk to a Friday evening when she had indeed taken the pill at 5:00 P.M. but by 5:40 she was vigorously vomiting the two beers and three shooters she'd sucked down during an unusually crazy happy hour.

Point to remember? The pill has to stay in your body to be effective, certainly more than a few minutes. The young woman in question was undoubtedly exaggerating her story, as missing only one pill in a cycle is unlikely to result in pregnancy. Typically, it would take more than a day or so before hormone levels drop to a point that could compromise effectiveness. But if two pills are missed in any one cycle, whether sequentially or at different times, a back-up method, like a condom, should definitely be used. I don't know if I was more incredulous at the amount of booze put away in a matter of moments or the fact that the young woman was resilient enough to continue with her Friday night revelry, concluding in a healthy dose of sex. Ah, the stamina of youth!

Can the pill help to regulate your periods?

Because you're taking a set amount of hormones with oral contraception, your menstrual cycle, including your period, will indeed become very regular. The artificial cycle controlled by the daily intake of synthetic hormones overrides your natural cycle. In fact, I can remember girls with whom I attended high school firmly stating that the only reason they were on the pill was to regulate their menstrual cycles or alleviate painful periods (dysmenorrhea). Obviously, such statements could only be met with disappointment and disbelief by pimply, adolescent walking penises, such as we were.

Can birth control pills be compromised by taking antibiotics?

Most definitely. When you go to the doctor's with some type of infection, like a strep throat, and the practitioner asks you, "Are you on any medications?" you need to answer in the affirmative. The pill is absolutely medication and antibiotics can lessen the pill's effectiveness against pregnancy. So, if you're on the pill and get prescribed antibiotics and you haven't discussed that fact with your practitioner, use a back-up method like a condom, just in case.

Can the pill reduce your sex drive?

Yes, isn't that a cruel irony. For some (definitely not all) women, an unwanted side effect of oral contraception is reduction or loss of libido (sex drive). But wait a minute, maybe that's why the pill is so effective, because you never want to have sex? Kidding, only kidding!

Does the pill have any positive side effects?

Yes indeed. In some women the pill will help reduce the incidence of acne; women who take the pill are less likely to develop ovarian or uterine cancer; some women find that the pill helps to reduce the development of benign breast lumps; and for women who have painful periods (dysmenorrhea) and/or endometriosis (where the lining of the uterus breaks away and can block the fallopian tubes), taking the pill can reduce the symptoms of these problems.

When are male contraceptive pills going to be available?

Does the expression "when hell freezes over" mean anything? When mountains crumble to the sea; when the oceans dry up; when the Washington Redskins win the Super Bowl again? Science has always been a male-dominated profession and if oral contraception seems to be working well for the women, why rock the boat? Besides, isn't it women and not men who get pregnant?

All joking aside, there is enough evidence to suggest that a male pill might be possible during this decade. Researchers continue to find various ways to decrease sperm motility, and such methods might be useful in committed relationships where the woman can trust the man to actually use the method. I don't see a future for this form of male pill in the singles world, where relationships are inevitably more casual and transient.

What's that new pill where you get fewer periods?

Until recently, when a woman who was taking the pill wanted to delay her period (maybe her "little monthly friend" was arriving on the eve of her wedding) the bride-to-be might throw away her final seven pills, which were essentially placebos anyway, open up a new pill pack and start on the active pills, thus delaying her period. This gave researchers an idea. Does a woman taking oral contraception need to have a period every month?

The answer is, probably not. The initial result of this thinking was Duramed's Seasonale, FDA approved in 2003. With this form of contraception, women take active pills for eighty-four days, followed by seven placebo pills, during which time the woman will menstruate. Do the math. This reduces the number of periods a woman experiences annually from the typical twelve to a much reduced four.

If you hate that little monthly visitor, this type of pill might be for you. Keep in mind, though, that like any of the oral contraception choices, many women may still experience some negative side effects that could include break-through bleeding or spotting, nausea, headaches, weight gain, mood swings, dizziness, and decreased libido. In 2006, Duramed introduced their latest extended regimen oral contraceptive, Seasonique, which also restricts periods to four a year, but with a shorter duration.

Is there a pill where you get no periods at all?

Wyeth has developed a pill called Lybrel that received FDA approval in June 2007. Lybrel is taken 365 days a year with no placebos, and therefore, no menstrual periods. So for those of you who want even fewer periods than Seasonale allows, Lybrel might be the answer.

What's up with those newer devices, the patch and the ring?

Think of the patch and the ring (NuvaRing) as pretty much the same as the pill, just different mechanisms of getting hormones into the body. Both these devices and the pill contain the combined hormones estrogen and progestin. These hormones work in the same way to prevent ovulation and thicken cervical mucus. The patch looks like a square Band-Aid and adheres to the skin (abdomen, buttocks, upper arm, or torso) and the hormones pass through the skin into the bloodstream. A single patch provides protection for seven days, then you replace it with another patch. Three consecutive patches prevent pregnancy for twenty-one days, and then the woman wears no patch for seven days, at which time she will menstruate. The ring also contains the two combined hormones, but unlike the patch, the ring is worn around the cervix for twenty-one days and then removed for seven. Choosing between these three similar methods is mainly predicated on the woman's preferences and habits.

Is "doubling up" on contraception with the pill and the condom an effective method?

It's a terrific method. Not only will the pill—if used correctly—provide almost foolproof protection against pregnancy, but the condom will also decrease the likelihood of your getting an STI. This combination is, next to abstinence, the most effective method of preventing both unintended pregnancy and STI transmission.

What is emergency contraception and how does it work?

Emergency contraception primarily consists of high-dose contraceptive pills. Because these are taken postintercourse, see the section on emergency contraceptive pills in the After Sex section, on page 119.

How good is Depo-Provera, commonly referred to as "the shot"?

The only injectable contraception currently available is Depo-Provera. This is a shot that is effective at preventing pregnancy for up to twelve weeks.

The shot contains only progestin, so women who don't tolerate the side effects caused by estrogen in the pill sometimes do better on Depo-Provera. This method is very effective, partly because it removes the possibility for user error or failure. In other words, you, the consumer, can't screw it up! There's no pill to forget, no condom to use incorrectly, no patch to forget to change, and no ring to insert incorrectly. As long as you get subsequent shots in time, pregnancy is virtually impossible.

Users will often cease menstruating, which concerns some women and delights others. Downsides include possible delayed fertility, increased weight gain and/or appetite, and Depo-Provera offers no protection against STIs.

During Sex

As a guy, what do I do to the clitoris when I find it?

Lesbians quite possibly make better lovers of women because they know all too well what feels good to the clitoris. Throughout the folklore of male sexuality, man has passed down the idea that when you finally stumble across the clitoris you should basically rub the hell out of it. I don't think so. Let's put this in terms that men can truly understand. Imagine someone gets hold of your very erect penis and vigorously rubs the heck out of its head! Feel good? After your eyes have finished watering and you've stopped crying I think we'll all agree that wasn't very pleasant. Think of the clitoris as a small organ that will respond much more readily to stroking along the shaft (side) and you'll find your attentions are much appreciated, and more effective.

That's a very large wet spot, so do women really ejaculate? And why?

Whenever I ask this question to the students in my course, most of them look bemused. But I can always rely on a few of the men, slouching back in their seats like the alpha-male gorilla pack, to nod knowingly, intimating that they of course have a very intimate knowledge of this very common occurrence. The crowd response is very different though, when the vivid technicolor film I use in class shows an inexplicable fluid spurting from the urethra of the woman energetically masturbating.

Female ejaculation is useful to consider as it symbolizes an important point—that despite incredible scientific advances in many fields, we clearly don't understand everything that occurs in human sexuality. I find that to be reassuring.

Some women seem to ejaculate, and we don't really know why. Longer answer: in the 1950s, gynecologist Dr. Ernest Grafenberg described a place on the anterior wall of the vagina that when stimulated could provide multiple orgasms, and the area was called the G-spot. Later, in the 1980s, researchers reported that some women who had their G-spot stimulated ejaculated a fluid from their urethras, in some cases quite forcefully.

Some women mistakenly think that because the fluid is released via the urethra they have lost bladder control and that the fluid is urine. That may be true in some cases, but in most, the fluid usually contains no trace of urine. The ejaculate is believed to originate in the woman's Skene's glands, and is often thought of as female prostatic fluid. However, there are no definite answers as to why some women ejaculate and others don't, and more specifically, the purpose of the fluid. Rest assured, it's not urine!

Can men have multiple orgasms?

Despite what you may have seen on the Internet or heard on the radio, there are no products that will provide men with multiple orgasms. I hate to burst the bubble for those of you who were charged $29.95 for a miracle product designed to keep you keepin' on, but you should get your money back. Despite some references in literature to men who have trained themselves to experience multiple orgasms (there is research to suggest that the Chinese were the first to be able to enjoy orgasm without ejaculation, thereby developing the potential for multiple orgasms), the harsh reality is that most men are not capable of multiple orgasms. When a man *fully* ejaculates, not pulls himself back from the edge of the abyss with slight leakage, then he enters what Masters and Johnson call the refractory period. At this postejaculatory stage, it doesn't matter what anyone does to the penis—sing to it, whistle to it, stroke it—it's not performing again until it takes a rest. The length of the rest period is dependent on several possible factors, most importantly the man's age.

If someone goes down on me, do I have to return the favor?

Ah, the etiquette of oral sex. Let's all admit to one thing: despite the expression that it is "greater to give than to receive," the vast majority of people prefer receiving to giving any day! So apart from the not-so-silent minority slurping themselves to heaven, most sex partners are faced with the postreception of fellatio or cunnilingus dilemma. Do I return the favor? My take on this is one of sheer politeness and sharing the wealth. Is it reasonable to ask someone to do something that you're not willing to do? The answer to this question is obvious to all fair-minded people, so take a deep breath, close your eyes, and get down there!

Some girls I'm with have a strong vaginal smell. How do I deal with this?

I'm always amazed by how many men are concerned with the "freshness" of a woman's nether regions while being totally oblivious to the rank odor emanating from their own stinking, unwashed genitalia. "What do you mean it smells? I had a shower just last week." Let me tell you, women's olfactory equipment is just as sensitive as yours, so any odor that you might generate is just as offensive to her nose.

The truth is that some women's vaginal odor may be stronger than others and isn't necessarily indicative of uncleanliness. My suggestion is, if you're going to be getting into oral sex and you know that ahead of time, suggest a little joint shower to get the ball rolling; that way both of you might be a little fresher.

After performing oral sex, my girlfriend wants to kiss me and that grosses me out. Am I being unreasonable not wanting my own stuff in my mouth?

I hear this question a great deal, and just as much from women. They too are not thrilled when the guy has been lapping at them like a parched golden retriever and then wants to plant a huge and extremely sloppy kiss on her mouth. Knowing that this concern is common to both sexes, I'd suggest a dramatic remedy—communicate! Tell your partner that you absolutely love it when he/she gives you orals, but that the prospect of sampling your own goods is less than a turn-on. (This despite the fact that most young adolescent males probably turned their bodies into pretzels trying to give themselves blow jobs before they finally found another person willing to save them from future back surgery.)

Will a woman's first time be painful?

The answer to this question depends on a number of factors. Pain can often occur because the woman's hymen is still intact and the hymen might be a little thicker or more firmly attached than is typical. Obviously, as the hymen tears due to the insertion of the penis, some pain would not be unusual. Another factor that might play a role is how nervous or anxious the individual is about having intercourse. Anxiety could reduce the volume of the female's vaginal lubrication, which in turn could lead to painful intercourse. How much sexual experience has the woman had prior to initial intercourse? If she has had a great deal of experience with "petting" (a professional term that sounds like you're stroking a German shepherd!) the woman may be much more relaxed when she has intercourse. In my research with college students, about one-third of women reported some level of discomfort and pain during their initial experience with penis-vagina intercourse.

Lights on or lights off?

Excellent question! If you were to believe all you see on television, you'd think that all sex not only occurred with the lights on, but with spotlights, cameras, reality television show hosts, and a panel of Lithuanian judges to score your performance. Let's be totally realistic, very few of us look incredible totally naked, and so the constant concern experienced by many individuals is, "What will the other person think when he/she first sees me naked?" Actually, let me rephrase that: "What will *he* think when *he* first sees me naked?"

Despite having some of the most repugnant and grossly shaped bodies ever to see the light of day, many men have such inflated egos that they simply don't care what their partner thinks. They know they're awesome, so what the hell? Women tend to be a bit more sensitive about their bodies and may be more likely to appreciate at least some muted lighting to enhance their features. This approach is less effective for men because they tend to be more visually oriented, and after spending their formative years masturbating themselves stupid in front of the computer screen or a glossy magazine, when they get themselves a real live human being with which to share their seed, they want to see and explore every nook and cranny, because who knows when they'll get this lucky again?

Ultimately, this question can only be answered through communication between partners. With the ever-increasing possibility that your naked picture will end up on someone's MySpace or YouTube page, maybe lights off is the better part of valor, at least until you can be sure that your lover isn't a part-time video producer. Work it, baby!

After sex, I usually use a vibrator to finish up. Do you think my boyfriend minds?

Not an uncommon scenario, but to be honest, I can't imagine your dragging out that vibrator after every sexual performance is doing much for boyfriend's self-esteem. It's kind of like, "OK, thanks for the foreplay, but seeing as you can't complete the deal I'm going to have to put my faith in my mechanical friend, the only lover on whom I can always rely to take care of business." Have you even talked about what goes on in bed (or doesn't) and how he feels about Battery Boy? One compromise might be to incorporate the vibrator into the entire act—that way you might climax with boyfriend actually participating in the process rather than listening to the relentless electronic buzz of the mechanical monster taking you to places boyfriend can only dream about.

I can't seem to ever get enough clitoral stimulation from either a partner or a vibrator. Can you suggest an alternative?

Actually, there is an electronic device that's about the size of a computer mouse and is specifically designed to stimulate the clitoris. It's called Eros-CTD, fits over the clitoris, and provides a gentle suction effect to increase blood flow and circulation. The device has been FDA approved, costs around $400, and is available in most countries without a prescription, but the United States requires a prescription to obtain this little device. Clearly the federal government is fine with facilitating orgasms as long as they're achieved for medical reasons.

In order to become aroused, I often feel the need to have a sexual fantasy before having sex with my boyfriend, and sometimes during sex too. Is this bad?

Fantasizing before and during sex is something just about everyone has done, but I'm not sure it's a piece of information you should freely offer up to your partner. I can just see your boyfriend looking into your eyes as you moan with delight and ask you what you're thinking about, and you breathlessly describe, without thinking, a scene involving a steamy shower room, oceans of foamy bubbles, and seven members of a college rugby team. Trust me, he won't take it well. Everyone has fantasized about sex at one time or another, so what you're experiencing is typical. I'd only be concerned about the issue if you compulsively require a fantasy *every* time you have sex.

It wasn't a fart, I swear—it was a queef!

So there you are, having great sex and loving life when all of a sudden the mood is broken by a loud ripping sound that can only be compared to a gut-busting fart. It's a bit of a shock the first time you hear it—she's shocked that he could rip one off at such a time, he's amazed that such a cute thing could sound like a truck driver, and yet in reality, the sound came from the vagina. It was a vaginal fart, air being trapped and released in the vagina from the thrusting motion of the penis. Some groovy person felt the need to invent a special word for this and so the term "queef," or "quefe," was born. Definitely makes it sound like a designer fart, doesn't it?

Whatever the hell you call it, should I just ignore it?

Sexual etiquette can be a tricky thing. If you make too big a deal of it you'll both become self-conscious and the mood will be ruined. On the other hand, if you're freaking out in case your partner thinks you really farted and want to clear that up once and for all, then maybe a brief conversation might be necessary. I think that if the "queefing" is only occasional, then you should just ignore it, but if it turns into a chronic problem where sex begins to sound like a third-grade boys' sleepover, then you'd better at least comment on it.

This issue is a great example of the need to have a sense of humor in the bedroom. If you and your partner can laugh about the queefing, you'll be fine. If all else fails, turn up the music good and loud.

Why does my boyfriend keep yelling nasty things while we're doing it?

Basically, because your boyfriend *is* nasty! Just kidding—well, maybe. What you have to remember is that everyone's sexual turn-ons are different and although there exists a kind of acceptable code of sexual behavior to which most folks adhere, there also exists a limitless array of possibilities for bedroom behavior. If your boyfriend gets off on yelling out crazy things while he's having sex, does it really matter? He could be doing things that would make the yelling of obscenities look like an afternoon on *Sesame Street*, so maybe this isn't so bad. Obviously, if this really bothers you, you'll need to talk to him about it. Try addressing him as a "goddamn, motherf****** son of a bitch" and see if he gets the point. Unfortunately for you, he might react by getting an erection, so be careful with this approach.

Do a lot of women really fake orgasms?

Does the sun come up in the morning? Is it cold in winter? Women faking orgasms is pretty common, just one of those things that you have to acknowledge as an integral part of life. And really, it doesn't have to be such a bad thing. A bold male student in one of my classes asked a general question, "How many of you women have faked an orgasm?" I was about to tell the women that they didn't have to respond, thinking that maybe the question was too personal, when 100 out of the 120 or so women present shot up their hands without hesitation! I wish I'd had a camera handy to record the male students' reactions as they did the math. I've never seen so many men simply lost for words.

But why do women fake it?

Men are easy. It takes all of a massive 2–5 seconds to become erect, and most men can ejaculate in under two minutes unless they try hard not to. Women take longer to vaginally lubricate and longer to climax, so Mother Nature has set up this tricky little heterosexual paradigm where a guy is constantly holding back and his female partner is constantly rushing forward, both hoping to meet somewhere in the middle, a magical, perhaps mythical place that can be very difficult to find, called *simultaneous orgasm.*

In addition, unlike men who can seemingly orgasm at the drop of a hat (or should that be panties?), many women are unable to orgasm every time they have intercourse, and although that might be an incomprehensible concept to most men, a large proportion of women are reconciled to this reality—it's just how it is.

Problems occur when men aren't aware of this concept or feel that they're not real men unless their partner climaxes. Guys with fragile egos don't like to hear, "I'm not coming today; it's me, not you!" And even really caring men who are holding back their orgasms so their mates can finally achieve climax don't get it that they might be on the job for literally days and still never reach an endpoint. A woman in my class, responding to the male question, "Why do women fake it?" replied, "To make it stop!"

So, some women, particularly those who might have someplace to be in the next five hours, find it easier to simply fake it rather than risk damage to the fragile male psyche or get into a lengthy harangue explaining why some women don't always have to orgasm every time.

So, is there an alternative to faking it?

I hate to repeat myself, but when a couple gets to know each other pretty well, both sexually and intimately, they usually feel comfortable being up-front about what's happening. Sometimes words aren't even necessary, so neither is faking it! When words are used, there's nothing wrong with the male asking his partner if she's "close" or if she's going to climax at all. At least the male will then have a much clearer idea of his immediate role and won't have the ignominious job of hammering away while his partner stares at the ceiling wondering whether or not to pull the fake.

Can a man tell when a woman is faking it?

In response to this question many of my male students nod knowingly, smirk a little, and sit back in their chairs, secure in the belief that they could never be fooled. Clearly this is a generation of self-absorbed men who've never seen "that" scene in *When Harry Met Sally*! A large majority of my female students admit to faking it at least once and in a large national study, where only 29 percent of women reported being able to orgasm every time during intercourse, 44 percent of men believed their partners climaxed every time. You do the math.

In one of my classes, the male students were asked to raise their hands if they were absolutely certain that a woman had never faked it with them. About fifty hands immediately shot up. As heads turned to recognize and acknowledge these self-appointed experts, a woman's voice from the other side of classroom punctured the air with, "Mike, you need to lower your hand right now—you've got to be kidding!" The other students howled and I don't think poor Mike returned to class for several weeks.

How many times can a person orgasm in an hour?

According to the Center for Marital and Sexual Studies in Long Beach, California the record number of orgasms witnessed in an hour was 16 for a male (impressive!) and 134 for a female. Come on, God has to be a woman. As amazing as those figures might seem, try to remember it's quality not quantity that counts, and being there in the moment is much more important than cranking out record-shattering numbers.

Is there an easy way to tell your partner that what he/she's doing isn't working for you?

The most important thing here is to avoid a totally negative response like, "Take your goddamn finger out of my butt, I hate that!" How about a more positive approach? Instead of saying what you *don't* like, how about getting to what you *do* like? Using the example above, this can be achieved by guiding your partner with your hands, gently removing your partner's offending digit from between your buttocks, and placing it somewhere else that might be more satisfying. Alternately, you could actually speak and say something like, "What I really like is" or, "I really like it when you . . ." You can suffer in silence for an eternity or be proactive and have much more pleasure. Doesn't seem like such a difficult choice, does it?

What sexual position tends to be the most satisfying for women?

That's kind of like asking what flavor of ice cream do women prefer. There are so many different preferences and opinions that there is no simple answer.

However, in the heterosexual world, the woman-on-top position gets rave reviews from most men and some women for some important reasons, none less crucial than the male has easy access to the clitoris and can stimulate this important little organ while intercourse proceeds. Remember that only a minority of women can orgasm from penis-vagina intercourse alone, so her male partner might need to give her a hand, if you see what I mean. Also, some women feel a little more in control on top and able to set the pace more effectively; in addition, the male is less likely to prematurely ejaculate on the bottom so that's clearly going to add to a woman's satisfaction.

Which positions do men and women seem to prefer?

In a 2007 *Esquire* and *Marie Claire* magazine survey of heterosexual sexual behavior, men's favorite sexual position was doggy style (man inserting penis into vagina from behind the woman) followed by woman on top, while women preferred missionary position with doggy style a second choice.

I can only orgasm when I'm on top of my boyfriend. Any tips for coming when I'm on the bottom?

A lot of women find orgasming on top easier than on the bottom. This has been ascribed to factors like the

woman being more in control of the pace and posi-
tioning, easier access for manual clitoral stimulation
during intercourse, and male partners lasting longer,
thus giving the woman more time to reach orgasm.
One obvious suggestion is to begin intercourse on
the top and when further down the road to climax,
switch positions to the bottom. Another tip is to communicate (dangerous, I know) that pressure on the
clitoris and pubic bone might be more effective for
you than the male thrusting his way to oblivion. Many
women report greater sexual excitement through
the pressure of the male's body on their clitoris rather
than through the man's athletic thrusting, that, while
quite impressive, is not as successful at accomplish-
ing clitoral stimulation.

What's up with guys wanting to rodeo all the time?

More recently, many of my female students have
commented that men today seem to enjoy having penis-vagina intercourse from behind a woman.
Most of the women seem to be cool with this, although some do complain about the lack of face-
to-face intimacy. The deal breaker for some women
though is their male partner's habit of slapping their
butts during the act, in an almost farcical rodeo
style . . . hence the development of the term "rodeo"
into a sexual verb. The sex-from-behind thing seems
quite popular now, but the rodeoing idea is a little

piece of male fantasy, incorporating what could be categorized as "disciplining" (see the Atypical Sexual Behavior section), where the male believes that most women basically enjoy being spanked. Although that might indeed be true for some women, I don't think the majority are up for that, and the women I spoke with were pretty pissed off about the whole thing.

Why do so many guys seem to be into anal sex?

An interesting trend that seems to be increasing recently is heterosexual anal sex. Most of the women who have spoken to me about this appear to be fairly indifferent but report that their male partners are seemingly hot for anal sex. Despite straight men in particular considering this a gay practice, sexuality research has long reported heterosexual anal sex as being fairly common, with as many as one in four having experienced this sexual delicacy. For many sexual partners this activity almost certainly speaks to curiosity, with perhaps a sense of adventure and the forbidden attached.

Interestingly, when I ask men in class what the attraction is with anal sex, all eyes immediately drop to the floor, feet shuffle nervously, and even the biggest self-anointed male studs simply refuse to acknowledge that they've visited that particular orifice. Unlike oral sex, about which men could discuss, analyze, and critique for hours, the average guy continues to feel very embarrassed about sexual contact in the "forbidden zone." Despite the trend of increasing heterosexual anal sex, the negative stigma remains firmly attached.

Does it mean anything if a guy doesn't kiss you during sex?

Maybe. I hate to be a total cynic, but let's be perfectly honest; to many men sexual intercourse is just another bodily function, and a female partner is just a depository for the fruits of that bodily function. Kissing is generally considered to be a very intimate activity and although the idea that kissing is more personal than oral sex or sexual intercourse might seem strange, many individuals adhere to that notion. Most men and women find kissing to be sexually arousing and so the idea that you would continue to kiss during intercourse would seem obvious. However, if the sex that is occurring is, shall we say "recreational" on the part of the male, he may be less inclined to perform the intimate act of kissing during intercourse. On the other hand, the male in question may love his partner dearly, but just not see kissing as part of his sexual lexicon beyond foreplay. One thing's for sure, the average male isn't famous for intimacy *after* he's done. So if you're not getting any kissing before *or* during sex, you might take that as a less than positive sign.

Is it OK to have sex with a woman while she's menstruating?

Some men can't stand the sight of blood and would be totally grossed out by the idea of sex with a menstruating woman, some men are indifferent and don't care either way, and some guys absolutely love it! A good friend in college who we'll call Dirty Dick, because basically that's how he was known, pretty much *only* had sex with women if they were menstruating. Despite spiraling laundry expenses, D^2 saw no problem with the practice and scoffed at any faint-hearted critics.

Despite being taboo in some cultures, there are no tangible reasons why a couple shouldn't have sex during the woman's period. In fact, there is evidence that in some cases, orgasms may relieve period pains and menstrual cramps.

If I have sex with my girlfriend during her period and we don't use any contraception, can she get pregnant?

The likelihood of a woman getting pregnant during her period is very slim, because she usually ovulates about fourteen days before her period and therefore there would be no viable egg present to be fertilized. However, if the woman happens to ovulate "off schedule" and near the time of menstruation (and you know, that would be just your luck) then it is possible that she could get pregnant. Always use a condom, just in case!

If you have sex from behind, is there a better chance you'll have a boy?

Ah, someone's been hearing about the Shettles' theory of sex selection! A certain Dr. L. B. Shettles, a fertility expert formerly from Columbia University, believes there are some things that you can do before and during intercourse to influence the sex of the baby you conceive. Male-bearing sperm seem to be more likely to perish in the acidic environment of the vagina, so according to Dr. Shettles, here's what you should do in order to maximize your chance of having a male child:

- Have intercourse immediately at the time of ovulation, so male-bearing sperm don't have to lie around getting wiped out waiting for the egg to make an appearance.
- Prior to intercourse the woman should have a baking-soda douche to produce a more alkaline and male-sperm-friendly environment.
- The sexual position should be one that provides the deepest penetration, thereby reducing the distance the male-bearing sperm has to travel, and that would be from behind, or "doggy" style.

How about if you want a girl? Dr. Shettles suggests:

- Have intercourse a day or so prior to ovulation, this way more male-bearing sperm will perish while waiting for the egg to arrive.
- Prior to intercourse the woman should have a dilute acetic acid (vinegar) douche to ramp up the acidity and make the environment less male-sperm friendly.
- The sexual position should be one that provides the shallowest penetration, thereby increasing the distance the male-bearing sperm has to travel, and that would be the missionary position, or man on top.

The likelihood of this system actually making any difference isn't great, but what do you have to lose? Only romance, perhaps. Not really very sexy, as you're hosing in the baking soda before being quickly nailed from behind. The things we do for children!

How long do the average male and female orgasms last?

The orgasm in both the male and female is the shortest phase of the human sexual response cycle—bummer! The average length of time for both genders to enjoy this magical moment is a mere ten seconds, although Masters and Johnson did document a forty-three second orgasm in one of their female subjects. And of course, women don't have to stop at one!

Why do some women make so much noise during sex, and others hardly any?

Just like some people are more exuberant about the ball game, chocolate cake, parties, or a movie, the same holds true for the bedroom. Both men and women will differ individually in how they respond sexually, with some panting and wailing at the slightest touch while others at the opposite end of the spectrum are so silent and still that you'd be worrying about necrophilia (that's sex with a dead person).

A college friend of mine was always visited by the same young lady on Wednesday evenings, a regular event marked by such howling and screaming that you'd think torture was occurring. My friend was only too happy to boast that his incredibly large penis was no doubt the reason for the woman's enthusiastic response—sure!

After Sex

Why do most guys seem to want to "flee the scene" three seconds after ejaculation?

This stereotypical male often considers sex, although very pleasurable, to hold little more importance than any other bodily function, like sneezing or peeing. Since the sex act holds no significance beyond the physical, when the man's done, he's done, and he goes about his business. Why should he stay? What else is there?

Now, in fairness, times do seem to be changing. Many men have realized that women actually have sexual needs and desires of their own, and although not necessarily acting out of intimacy but rather to be viewed as a man who "can get the job done," these men are breaking the three-second barrier and hanging out longer. Also, in a time where many young women pride themselves on "hooking up", without complications, perhaps we are seeing a shift where women don't want men to hang around longer than necessary anyway, or perhaps it's the woman who takes her pleasure and is back on the road in seconds.

If I don't call a girl after having sex, will she think I've just used her or is it cool?

It depends. Ever think *she* might have used *you*? This is an interesting question as it suggests that little or no communication occurred before or after the deed. Was this a one-night stand? Had you been seeing her for a while, or had you been talking prior to having sex? Was there any spoken intention to see each other again? You get the idea. There are so many "it depends" that this question is impossible to answer. In a modern world where there seems to be an increase of young women casually hooking up, I think the answer would be that perhaps no one really thinks anything of it.

How likely is it that I'd get pregnant if we didn't use contraception?

With my tongue firmly in cheek, I'd say there's undoubtedly an inverse relationship between how much you don't want to be pregnant and the odds of getting pregnant! Obviously, the odds of your getting pregnant will be higher if you've had intercourse around the time you ovulate. However, taking the month as a whole, if we agree that sperm is viable for about three days, and we use this three-day window period to estimate risk, the odds of getting pregnant from a one-time sexual encounter, at first glance, are roughly 10 percent. But, just to muddy the waters, because some medical experts estimate that conception only occurs about 25–50 percent of the time that sperm actually meet an ova, the odds of pregnancy from one-time sex could be reduced to around 3–5 percent. Now, don't go and use this as a feeble excuse not to use contraception. The odds of your getting pregnant if you absolutely, positively, really don't want to get pregnant are more like 100 percent. It's Murphy's Law.

What if I don't lose my hard-on after having sex? How quickly should it go away?

An erection that lasts for over four hours, and has not been maintained through sexual stimulation, is called priapism. The most common cause of this condition is a response to medications, including some antidepressants. Also, since the introduction of those little blue wonder pills—Viagra and their kind— a reported side effect for a small percentage of men is prolonged erection. Although a perpetual boner might sound like every man's dream, the condition can be dangerous, to say nothing of downright em- barrassing.

Priapism occurs when blood flows into the erectile

tissue of the penis (corpora cavernosa and corpus spongiosum) but not out. Because the blood is no longer circulating, the erectile tissue is deprived of oxygen, resulting in an erection that can be painful and, if not treated, can result in permanent damage to the functionality of the penis. The treatment isn't a lot of fun. Let's just say it involves needles and removal of the offending blood and leave it at that. This side effect is something to remember for any of you playboys who might be using Viagra for recreational purposes.

Why is it that sometimes after sex I can get an erection almost immediately and go again, while at other times I'm done for the night?

Here's another of those "it depends" answers. Some of the reasons may be tangible and therefore predictable. Why might you get another erection very quickly? Well, maybe you've just ended a dry spell and after years of chronic masturbation you finally have someone other than your right hand with you in your bed. Others could be that you find your partner astonishingly sexy; you're really into your partner; you're watching porn; you're watching someone else watching porn. You get the idea, it could be one of several factors.

Reasons why you might be done for the night: you're smashed and were lucky to be able to have sex once; you're exhausted after running the Boston

Marathon that morning; you really don't like your partner that much; you're stressed out over something; or you forgot to rent the porn. Most of the time, you'll never know the reason for your sad lack of tumescence—you'll just have to put it down to biorhythms and live with it.

What determines the length of the refractory period?

Just a refresher: the refractory period refers to the time postejaculation, when no matter what you do to the penis, it will not respond to sexual stimulation. The most influential factor for this period tends to be the man's age. Clearly, a seventeen-year-old boy will have a much shorter refractory period than a seventy-year-old man. Of course, the seventeen-year-old boy will most likely have prematurely ejaculated in seconds anyway, so why would his penis need much of a rest? Other factors could also be drinking too much, fatigue, illness, or how long it's been since the last time you ejaculated.

Why do only men have the refractory period?

Because, my friend, like I said earlier, God is a woman! She has to be. Why else would women have the potential to just keep pumping out orgasms like a machine while men shrink to a shadow of their former selves and have to sit around waiting for their erection to return? In a procreative sense, there is a theory that because it takes men approximately seventy-two hours to restock their sperm bank, so to speak, what would be the point of their having intercourse again when their sperm levels would be pathetic and most likely ineffective? A woman looking to procreate would need to move on to another man who could provide her a full amount of sperm. It's a theory, but I still think God's a woman.

My boyfriend is very affectionate with me and tells me that he loves me, but after we've had sex it's like he's another person and he barely speaks to me. What's up with that?

What's up with that? Your boyfriend is a self-centered, self-absorbed, egocentric, selfish lover who could care less about your feelings. In other words, he's a male. Some men would argue that they are wired such that when they've ejaculated, some mysterious hormone is released that commands them to shut down all physical and verbal communication with their partner. Others claim that socialization has brainwashed them into being less intimate and sharing lest they be perceived as weak and vulnerable. One thing's for sure, it's not the guy's fault. He's a victim of his biology and/or culture. You make the call.

What's up with the morning-after pill and does it really work?

Emergency contraceptive pills are intended for use by women who had sex without using any contraception, or whose partner's condom broke, and are used as a means to decrease the likelihood of becoming pregnant. Years before the FDA approved a prepackaged emergency contraception pill pack in 1998, practitioners had opened oral contraception pill packs to give a woman some magic number of pills and then thrown away the remainder. This was obviously very wasteful and expensive. The most commonly used emergency contraceptive pills (ECP) currently on the market are appropriately called Plan B. The pills contain progestin-only medication, and despite its "morning-after" title, this method is thought to be effective if taken up to seventy-two hours after the time of risky activity (and some researchers believe that window of opportunity could be as long as 120 hours). Another product called Preven is also available; this type of pill contains progestin and estrogen. Effectiveness rates are difficult to calculate since no one knows whether or not the egg was ever fertilized in the first place, nor how many women would have actually become pregnant, but they are estimated to be 75 percent for Preven and 89 percent for Plan B. Both types of pill can cause unpleasant side effects, including very bad nausea, so some practitioners will provide a woman with an antinausea drug along with the emergency contraceptive pills.

So how does ECP actually work?

Most experts believe that ECP works by interfering with the fertilization and implantation of an egg and not by causing any type of abortion. Obviously, a constituency exists that disagrees and considers this method of contraception to be the same as an abortion.

Couldn't I just use ECP as my method of contraception when I'm having sex?

Absolutely not. This method is intended to be a backup for when Rambo breaks that condom, or when you both get too drunk to remember what a condom is. Effectiveness rates are not as good as using oral contraception or Depo-Provera, plus you have the nasty side effects to consider. So, no, this shouldn't be used as your regular method of contraception.

Where can you get emergency contraceptive pills?

You used to only be able to get these pills from your medical provider or clinic, but in 2006 the FDA finally broke down and permitted access to ECP as an over-the-counter (OTC) medication, available from pharmacies. Despite two expert scientific panels basically stating that ECP was safer than an aspirin, the FDA, under transparent pressure from the White House, initially refused to allow OTC status for this medication. Even after OTC status was grudgingly provided, it came with a huge caveat—it's only available to women over 18 years of age. I mean, come on, we don't want to make it available to the people who really need it, do we? Compared to older females, younger women, and teens in particular, use contraception less often and less effectively, and are therefore in greater need of access to ECP. Yet another sublimely appropriate example of how human sexuality is more about politics than it is about getting physical—or even about common sense, come to that!

Why do people say women should urinate immediately after sex?

Some people have suggested that if a woman urinates immediately after vaginal intercourse she may be able to flush out any bacteria that have found a home in her urethra during sex. The presence of such bacteria might result in a urinary tract infection (UTI) that can be treated with antibiotics. This advice should go down in the "it probably won't make a difference, but it can't hurt" column.

PART THREE

The Other Stuff

It's Just a Little Rash:
Sexually Transmitted Infections
(STIs)

When I look at my two hundred or so students as I begin my unit on sexually transmitted infections (STIs), I make the statement that according to reported data from college campuses, about 30–40 of them have had or currently have a sexually transmitted infection. There is a tense, awkward moment as the students twist their heads around in a vain attempt to identify the poor bastards who have the infections. Each student is sure of only one thing—that he or she doesn't have one!

I've often considered hiring a ringer, a student who would leap out of her seat at this point, passionately screaming out, "Listen to him, listen to Dr. Sawyer, what he's telling you is true. I have herpes, I really do. Actually, it's a raging case of herpes and you need to know this is for real." But of course this is only a fantasy, and as I look at the students' faces I can see they don't think this is their problem. Unfortunately, it most definitely is.

Adolescents aged 18–24 account for the highest proportion of cases for all STIs. In fact, STIs are at pandemic levels on nearly all university and college campuses, and of all the sexual problems to which a student might fall prey, getting an STI is the most likely.

Sexually transmitted infections have been around forever. The common theme with all these diseases is the seemingly out of control need to blame someone else for them. During the times of global exploration and colonization, Europeans blamed the natives for infecting the pure and virtuous visitors to their shores, who then took the diseases back to Europe to continue the epidemic. The natives of course blamed the explorers for bringing the pox to the pristine shores of the New World.

Later in history, when Europe was ravaging itself in the Hundred Years War, the French called syphilis the Spanish disease, the Spanish called it the English plague, the English of course blamed the French, and so on and so on. Little was understood about these types of infections and, in fact, even as science progressed through the centuries, knowledge continued to be very limited.

No better example illustrates this fact than the infamous mistake made by English physician, Dr. John

Hunter in 1767. He self-inoculated himself with gonor-rhea from a patient, not knowing the man was also infected with syphilis. When he developed both infec-tions, Dr. Hunter incorrectly announced that they were the same disease.

Today we don't blame entire nations; we just blame each other. After working for many years in a college sexual health clinic, I can anticipate a patient's reac-tion to a diagnosis of infection by their gender. Women react to the news of their infection with embarrass-ment, guilt, shame, regret, and all too frequently, with tears. Men simply respond, "*She* gave me this. I can't believe she'd do this to me." Although the facts tell us that women are more likely to get an STI from a man than vice versa, spending twenty years of working with collegiate infections could make a person think a man has never given an infection to a woman.

Let's get the names and definitions out of the way. Until the 1960s, the two most dreaded letters in the En-glish language were VD (venereal disease). Reaction to these two little letters was visceral. Such was the neg-ative stigma surrounding these letters that they were al-ways spoken of in hushed terms, almost a superstitious whisper, as if saying them too loudly would guarantee an infection.

In the seventies the terminology for "VD" was re-placed with "sexually transmitted diseases" or "STD," referring to a series of diseases that were sexually trans-missible. Finally a few years ago, federal health agen-cies determined that "disease" sounded too severe, so to lessen anxiety they suggested a change to sexually transmitted "infections."

Well intended, but ludicrously naïve—do they honestly think that some freaked-out adolescent will feel better because they could say, "It's okay, it's just a teensy little *infection*?" Quite frankly, if you've got an infection of the genitals, I don't think you give a damn about semantics, you just want to get treated! So these days you will usually see either of the two acronyms STDs or STIs. They can be used interchangeably, though I suspect you don't want any reason to use either of them!

Who's at greater risk for STIs, men or women?

Women have it worse than men when it comes to STIs for a few reasons. A woman's vagina provides a large surface area and an environment that is conducive to the growth of pathogens. Males have a narrow tube called a urethra inside the penis, so there's a much smaller surface area on which to grow bacteria or viruses. Also, men ejaculate into women, and along with the semen ride the bacteria and viruses, while women tend not to ejaculate into the penis.

How soon will I get symptoms after someone gives me a sexually transmitted infection?

Short answer: If you're a woman, you may never get symptoms and you wouldn't know you were infected until your male partner tells you; your infection is detected by routine screening like a gynecological exam; or you develop a secondary infection like pelvic inflammatory disease (PID). Males traditionally have symptoms, but the length of time before the symptoms appear are disease specific and can be long and unpredictable.

How can you tell if someone has an infection?

It's almost impossible. Most men who have some pretty obvious symptoms aren't going to want to have sex anyway, so they tend to be out of the picture. Most women have few or no symptoms, so, again, detection is a real problem. Stereotypically, most men get diagnosed at a clinic after having obvious symptoms checked, while many women who haven't been told by a sexual partner that they might have an infection are diagnosed through a routine screening, like a pelvic exam.

So how do you prevent STIs?

You've probably heard of some pretty weird answers to this question. "Ask someone if he or she has an infection." Oh, right, that'll work. "Would you like a Heineken, and do you have herpes, or anything?" I can assure you, no sexual contact will *ever* follow that question. I also hear, "Ask your partner about his or her previous partners." I can just see a guy pulling out a flow chart of past partners at the bar. Talk about a mood breaker! And how much meaningful information could you really gather? Not much.

Ann Landers, in one of her newspaper columns, advised, "Before having sex with a new partner, always inspect their genitalia!" Who feels comfortable stark naked in front of a new partner? Sex in our culture tends to occur under the sheets with the lights off, so you'd better get that nightscope out. Didn't we just say that women have no symptoms? A man could explore her entire depths with a mining helmet and a wet suit and find nothing. Dumb!

I've also heard, "Immediately upon ejaculation the man should urinate"—the rationale being that he could maybe flush out those unwanted bugs. First, this does nothing to improve the image of men's total lack of postcoital intimacy. Second, which man on this planet can urinate with an erection? Men have this damn problem every morning of their lives, waiting for their tumescence to point at the porcelain, not at the ceiling—very inconvenient.

If you didn't already know, none of these methods is effective.

So really, how do you prevent STIs?

The only 100 percent effective method is abstinence. Outside the church, it's not a really popular method (although it is absolutely foolproof and for some, worth considering). The next best thing is to find a person who will be your only sex partner, and he or she will do the same for you. That's called monogamy. If neither of you is bringing an infection into the relationship, then you won't ever get an STI. Caution, do not confuse this with serial monogamy; thirteen monogamous relationships a year doesn't count. Finally, the only method of contraception that provides effective protection against nearly all STIs is a latex condom.

Can you get more than one STI at a time?

You can be infected by as many different diseases with which you come into direct contact. On one occasion, while working in an STI clinic, I saw a person with as many as five different infections.

Can you get these infections orally?

"You can get something wherever you put something" is the STI adage I give my students. It's hardly Shakespeare, but I think you get my drift. For example, chlamydia can be found in the penis, rectum, and vagina, while gonorrhea can be found in all those places plus the throat.

Is it possible to get an STI without having sex?

Here it comes, a man seeking an alibi for a misspent Saturday night! The short answer to your question is, you *could* contract some STI without having had sex, but the likelihood is about the same as your winning the lottery. Here's the familiar story I would hear in the campus clinic: A male student's girlfriend had gone home for the weekend, and so quite understandably—with sex being kind of like oxygen, you know, a necessity for survival—the boyfriend had extracurricular sex on Saturday night. When the girlfriend returned on Sunday night, the male student had to welcome her with rampant sex, pretending he hadn't gotten any for forty-eight hours. On Wednesday, he gets the telltale symptoms of gonorrhea and reports to the clinic in search of penicillin and an alibi, a way he must have become infected that didn't involve another human being, you know, a doorknob or toilet seat, maybe? Sorry guy, there's pretty much only one way to get gonorrhea. It's honesty time.

So you can't get an STI off a toilet seat?

Actually, believe it or not, a study was performed to see if gonorrhea could be cultured off a toilet seat, and here's what was projected. If you stand outside a public restroom, with your pants down and in a sprint start position, and as soon as the door opens you hurl yourself into the restroom, immediately rubbing your penis or vagina all over the toilet seat, it's still almost impossible to contract gonorrhea. And let me tell you, if you're rubbing your nether regions all

x

over the vile surface of a public toilet seat, then you deserve any disease you get.

How about the incubation periods of infections?

With the exception of gonorrhea (which has a very short incubation period), most infections have incubation periods that range from 21–30 days. However, there are a few infections, including chlamydia and HPV, that seem to buck the system. Although most sources will give you the standard 21–30 days incubation period for nearly all STIs, there is sufficient evidence to suggest that with some infections, the incubation period can be much longer.

The social problems that this can cause are profound. You've been seeing the same person exclusively for a few months and just started to have sex with that person when suddenly you've got some symptoms. You know that you haven't been running around, but now you're questioning how well you really know this person and whether or not they've been cheating with half your circle of friends. A million scenarios run through your mind as your emotions change wildly from sadness to fantasies about physical violence with a sharp object.

Here's the truth: unless one of you was a virgin on entering the relationship, determining who gave what to whom is almost an impossibility. (Of course, this does not take into account the universal maxim of man never infecting woman in the history of the world, but in the interest of truth, we'll let that slide for the moment.) Your partner may have brought the infection into the relationship asymptomatically, and only upon having sex with you, passed on the infection. For that matter, maybe you contracted the infection from a previous partner and have only just started to exhibit symptoms and now possibly infected your new partner. All these are important points to consider before pulling out the machete and reconfiguring your partner's better features.

What are the most common STIs that young adults are likely to get?

The two most common STIs in the 16–35 age group are chlamydia and human papilloma virus (HPV, which can cause genital warts).

So what's the deal with the virus that causes genital warts? Is it serious?

A virus that was barely recognized by the public only a few years ago has almost become a house-hold name today. Genital warts is pretty much at epidemic levels, particularly in the young-adult age groups. For men, genital warts are unsightly, embar-rassing, and altogether unpleasant, but for women the stakes are much higher. Because this particular little bug is a nasty one, we need to take a little time to understand it better, so take a close look at the information that follows, despite the fact, of course, that *you* would never get an STI!

The Most Common STIs

Human Papilloma Virus (HPV)—and Genital Warts

Here are the numbers. According to the Centers for Disease Control (CDC), approximately twenty million people in the United States are currently infected with HPV. At least 50 percent of sexually active men and women acquire genital HPV infection at some point in their lives. By age fifty, at least 80 percent of women will have acquired genital HPV infection. About 6.2 million more Americans get a genital HPV infection each year. These are pretty powerful numbers, and this is becoming a really common infection. For women in particular. HPV can lead to serious consequences. so read this section carefully.

HPV has become one of the most common infections in the 18–35 age group and consists of over one hundred types of the virus. Some of the viruses are known as "high risk" because they can result in abnormal Pap smears and increase the likelihood of developing cervical cancer. Although the odds are that a woman who contracts HPV will have no symptoms, will not develop cervical cancer, and in fact the virus will become dormant without treatment, in some cases the virus can lead to precancerous cell growth in the cervix. Some women develop warts that are visible, but many women who are infected have no symptoms. It's important to remember that the types of HPV that cause genital warts are thought to be different from the types that cause cervical cancer.

The vast majority of HPV is diagnosed through an abnormal Pap test often accompanied or followed by a test for the presence of HPV DNA. The most common treatment of HPV in women is cryotherapy, where the tissue around the cervix is frozen. Women who have been diagnosed with genital warts should have pelvic exams and Pap smears at least once a year.

What about the men?

The CDC estimates that around 50 percent of sexually active men will have HPV at some point in their lives. Right now, there is no practical test for HPV in men. For the most part, a visual inspection of the genitalia and anus can be performed to look for the presence of genital warts. Some practitioners apply a dilute solution of acetic acid (yes, men, that's vinegar—we're pickling the penis!) to the shaft of the penis and then use a very bright light to look for white, subcutaneous patches that might be HPV. This area, in addition to any warts that might be visible without the acetic acid, can be treated with a solution called podophyllin that will remove the warts after one or two treatments. Visible warts can also be frozen off or surgically removed, but the virus will still be present in the body. Most men obviously want the warts removed from the penis, however, removing the warts is no guarantee that HPV will not be transmitted. The medical consequences of HPV for men are much less serious than for women, so the ability to transmit the virus from a man to a woman is probably the most troubling concern.

How about immunization against HPV?

Although there's no real cure for HPV, in 2006 the FDA approved pharmaceutical company Merck's vaccine, Gardasil. This three-injection immunization will protect women against HPV strains 16 and 18 (that are responsible for about 70 percent of all cervical cancer), in addition to strains 6 and 11 (that cause about 90 percent of genital warts). The shots are recommended for females aged 12–26 who have not come into contact with the virus, although some experts are suggesting that even women who have been infected would benefit from the immunization as they are unlikely to have been infected with all four strains of the virus.

Won't this encourage more young girls to have more sex?

Who started the myth that information and protection increase sexual behavior? Let me see if I understand the rationale. A twelve-year-old girl who gets immunized against a virus that she probably can't even pronounce, never mind spell, will suddenly become promiscuous at fourteen because of the knowledge that her risk for cervical cancer is diminished? This mental meandering defies belief and understanding. Here we have an incredible medical breakthrough that can potentially decrease cervical cancer rates by 70 percent and the moral conscience of the country is more concerned with the theoretical sexual behavior of teens—please! Thankfully, common sense is prevailing with many school jurisdictions mandating HPV vaccination as a requirement for school attendance.

Chlamydia

Chlamydia has become one of the most common STIs in young adults with an estimated three million new cases a year in the U.S. It is so common in young women that by the age of thirty about half of all sexually active women have been infected with chlamydia. Chlamydia can be transmitted through vaginal, anal, or oral intercourse, so for those of you folks continuing to convince yourselves that licking a person's genitalia is perfectly safe and has no connection to sex, you'd better pay attention! The vast majority of women have no symptoms for this infection, and even about 50 percent of men can be asymptomatic. If a woman has symptoms, she is likely to experience burning during urination and pain during intercourse. Men tend to experience a rather watery discharge and discomfort urinating.

In women, testing has become more routine as part of the pelvic exam, which is just as well, given that most women have no symptoms and a huge number of infections would go unnoticed without the pelvic exam.

A culture is usually performed, although blood tests are also available.

In men, a urine test is available, making unnecessary an earlier procedure of using a type of long Q-tip to explore the depths of the urethra to search for offending pathogens. Although the urine test is probably much more efficient, I feel it doesn't quite capture the imagination and attention that the old Q-tip could, perhaps lingering in the victim's, I mean *patient's,* memory the next time he's about to be too cavalier to slip into a condom.

In many clinic settings, males are diagnosed with a "catch all" term called nongonococcal urethritis (NGU). They are tested for gonorrhea, and if the test comes back negative but there are many white blood cells present, then the man is diagnosed with an infection of the urethra that simply isn't caused by gonorrhea—NGU.

Treatment for chlamydia, for both men and women, is usually a course of antibiotics, such as tetracycline or doxcycline, for seven to ten days. If the infected person has a current sexual partner, he or she should be treated at the same time, or the infection will come bouncing back. Nontreatment for men infected with chlamydia could lead to epididymitis (an infection in the organs that store immature sperm in the testes) that can cause your testes to swell and ache—not much fun, but usually not too serious.

Women who are not treated, on the other hand, may develop pelvic inflammatory disease (PID), where the tiny and fragile fallopian tubes through which the woman's eggs travel can become infected and swollen. Although PID can be successfully treated with antibiotics, the buildup of scar tissue can cause infertility, a high price to pay for an untreated STI.

Given the asymptomatic nature of chlamydia, my advice would be that if you are a woman who has had penis-vagina intercourse in the past three months and a condom wasn't used, you should get a chlamydia culture now. Better safe than sorry.

Can lesbians get chlamydia?

Absolutely. Oral sex and vulva-to-vulva contact can transmit chlamydia. And don't forget that women are less likely to have symptoms anyway, so two people together where neither is likely to have a symptom could mean a real risk of transmission. Also, some people at a young age might have experimented with heterosexuality before beginning a same-gender relationship.

Gonorrhea

This disease has been around for centuries and at one point was probably the most common STI in the world. That was long before the more recent infections like HPV and chlamydia came along, relegating poor old gonorrhea to a less lofty place on the hit parade of infections. Nevertheless, gonorrhea can still claim a healthy 650,000 new victims in the U.S. each year, not a bad number for a disease on the wane! Long known by the slang term of clap (possibly named after *les clapiers,* the buildings Parisian prostitutes lived in), this infection is caused by a bacteria that thrives in the mucus membranes of the body—urethra, vagina, anus, mouth, and throat. Once again, you oral experts need to take note.

The incubation period for gonorrhea is one of the fastest in this group of infections, anywhere from 2–8 days. Women often have no symptoms for this infection but if they do, the symptoms include vaginal bleeding, unusual vaginal discharge, and an increase in urinary frequency. Males usually experience a thick, whitish discharge, with a burning sensation during urination, that some have described as feeling like "peeing through broken glass"! Not a lot of fun. If individuals have had oral and/or anal sex, those sites could also become infected and would need to be tested for infection.

Until recently, the most typical type of test was to use a cotton swab to obtain a sample of any discharge from around the penis for men and the cervix for women in order to run a culture test. A less invasive urine test is now available. A gram stain test can also be performed quickly by examining a sample of the discharge under a microscope. Treatment for both men and women involves the use of an antibiotic, such as ceftriaxone. But because some strains have become resistant to antibiotics, the person should be examined about a week after treatment to make sure that the infection has been cured.

Herpes

Herpes simplex virus 2 (HSV-2), the bug that causes genital herpes, is part of a large family of herpes viruses, including that typically adolescent problem of mononucleosis and the childhood disease of chicken pox. See, you had no idea that you've already had herpes. "No, wait!" I hear you cry, "I haven't had *that* type of herpes, just a little childhood infection!"

Don't get too excited. What you don't realize is that you probably have been exposed to herpes, with estimates of as many as 80 percent of adult Americans infected with HSV-1 (more commonly known as cold sores), with about one-third of these folks experiencing symptoms. Rates of HSV-2 (genital herpes) in the American population are estimated to be one in five, so you see, the odds are that you have the "real" herpes anyway!

Herpes tends to be a good news/bad news scenario. The bad news is that although huge proportions of sexually active people seem to carry the virus, the good news is that much smaller numbers of them actually have outbreaks. But then again, some more bad news suggests that although some people don't have symptoms, they can still pass on the infection to another person, so I suppose on aggregate there's more bad news than good.

HSV-1 VERSUS HSV-2

"I don't really have herpes; it's just a cold sore!" The generalized difference between HSV-1 and HSV-2 is that number 2 is found below the belt (genitally) and number 1 is found above the belt (cold sore). Although the DNA of the two viruses are fractionally different, their similarities are mimicked by the parallel development of symptoms.

Whether on the labia, penis, or lip, the person will feel a tingling feeling in the area, a small bump will appear that gradually gets larger as the volume of fluid under the skin grows, and after a couple of days the skin will break open, giving the person an incredibly attractive open and bloody sore. The sores can be very painful and will last for approximately 8–10 days. Let's just say the chance of your getting a date with this lovely looking sore on your lip, never mind your genitalia, is usually in inverse proportion to your total embarrassment and humiliation.

After what seems like an eternity, the offending scab will fall off and your appearance will return to its pristine condition, until the next time. Unfortunately, there is an excellent chance that there will be a next time, but fortunately, as you age, your body seems to develop some immunity that gradually inhibits the number of future outbreaks. That said, the progression is identical for HSV-1 and -2, so to me if they look the same, sound the same, and smell the same, they may as well be one and the same.

Going on a field trip?

To make the difference between viruses 1 and 2 an even more irrelevant point, let's consider the migration of the virus from one area to another. Let's just suppose that to avoid all the nasty stuff that can occur from penis-vagina sex a couple decides to "play it safe" by just getting down to some good old oral sex. The woman goes down on the guy and gives him a hummer of vast proportions, but because he has no symptoms yet, the woman doesn't realize that her partner has HSV-2. We'll keep the story simple (and realistic) as the male fails to reciprocate.

A few days later the woman feels a bump on her lip, and sure enough she experiences an outbreak of herpes—but of what type? Surely her lip is way above her belt, so shouldn't she have HSV-1? Look, the virus that she contracted doesn't pop out of her lip and exclaim, "This doesn't look like a vagina. I must have morphed into a number 1 virus." The cold sore now being experienced by the oral lover has been caused by HSV-2, though of course she's entitled to claim, "It's just a cold sore!"

By the same process in reverse, a person who has HSV-1 can transmit that virus to someone's genitals through oral sex, but the virus will remain number 1, and knowing all this, does anyone really care about the number?

How do you test for herpes?

Testing is usually done by taking some cell samples from the blisters, so diagnosis is really helped by having a symptom. In my time working in an STI clinic I would see male after male who would tell me they had "something" on their penis about two months ago and it's gone now . . . what did I think it was?! Oh, damn, I forgot my crystal ball—how would I freaking know what he had? It could have been herpes but it could just as easily have been a zit! The message here is loud and clear—*go and get checked out when you have something to check!* There are blood tests available, but all they can tell you is whether or not you've been exposed to the virus, not whether you'll have any outbreaks. Given that half the population has been exposed, I'm not sure of the value of that particular test.

Vaginitis

Vaginitis? If we're talking infection of the vagina, this doesn't concern men, right? That would be a true statement if the vast majority of men didn't have an almost compulsive desire and need, to get close to, near to, or get inside a vagina. Because of this "connection," men can be infected with forms of vaginitis and can also infect women. If you're a woman who is repeatedly getting vaginal infections and your sexual partner (male or female) has not been checked and/or treated, then he or she could be the source of your very annoying reinfections!

Yeast infection (moniliasis, candidiasis)

There are many different forms of vaginal infections, one of the most common being a yeast infection. And finally, yes, *this* is an infection that you can get without ever having had sex. Most women at some point in their lives will have a yeast infection. This is basically a fungal infection, and for women the symptoms may include one or more of the following: a cottage-cheese–like vaginal discharge, an itchy feeling in the vagina, redness on the labia, and a burning feeling. Treatments include over-the-counter vaginal suppositories or creams that usually take a few days to work, and there is also an available oral medication. Individuals can use a one-day treatment but some practitioners are concerned that the one-day regimen might not completely cure the infection.

Men, being men, know yeast infections by the term "jock itch." This is a fungal infection of the skin that results in a red, itchy rash often found on the shaft of the penis, the scrotal sac, and most likely the V where the legs meet the body's trunk. Treatment is usually an over-the-counter cream like Lotrisone, with a recommendation to keep the affected area dry with talcum powder. Yes men, you can actually get this infection without being an athlete, and most disappointingly, without having sex.

Trichomoniasis

This little beauty is caused by a protozoa, a single-celled parasite that can be transmitted during penis-vagina intercourse and also from woman-to-woman genital contact. The symptoms in women are pretty unpleasant: a greenish, frothy, vaginal discharge with a bad odor that occurs around 5–28 days after exposure. Males can experience some mild discharge and some men have described the symptom as having an itch in the middle of their penis that they can't scratch.

The treatment for this infection is an oral antiparasitic medication called Flagyl that has some very nasty side effects should you drink alcohol while on this prescription. Can you say violent vomiting? This infection can possibly be transmitted without having had sexual contact, such as if two women were to share a bikini bottom or underwear that had been previously worn by an infected person.

Pelvic Inflammatory Disease (PID)

Pelvic inflammatory disease (PID) is a general term that refers to an infection of the uterus and fallopian tubes, most often caused by the STIs chlamydia and gonorrhea. In the United States there are about one million cases of acute PID annually, and each year PID causes approximately 100,000 women to become infertile.

The STI travels through the vagina, the uterus, and into the fallopian tubes, and if untreated, PID can result in symptoms like an unusual vaginal discharge, abdominal pain, bleeding after sex, or perhaps worse, no symptoms at all.

Pelvic inflammatory disease can be difficult to diagnose, and unfortunately, sometimes by the time a diagnosis is made, permanent damage has occurred. Although antibiotics can cure the infection, because of scarring or damage to the lining of the fallopian tubes, some cases of PID will result in infertility.

How can I prevent PID?

Always use a condom when having vaginal inter-course, at least until you're absolutely 1,000 percent certain that your partner hasn't brought you some undiagnosed souvenir from his last relationship. Basically, if you can greatly reduce the risk of contracting an STI, you'll also have way less likelihood of developing PID. (Why have these bad things all got three letters?) Also, if you're a woman, who for whatever reason had vaginal sex without your partner using that magic latex protection, you should go and get tested for possible STI infection rather than wait eight months for your next pelvic exam, by which time PID could be wreaking havoc. I can't stress enough the danger to women. Remember, you will probably have no symptoms for STIs, so how would you even know that PID might develop? Again, the answer is to get yourself a checkup if you ever have vaginal sex without a condom. Not doing that could be very costly.

The Plague of the Century:
HIV/AIDS

There was a time in the 1960s and 1970s when the most feared sexually transmitted disease on college campuses was herpes. *Time* magazine heralded the high prevalence of this disease with a lengthy article and a large H became the scarlet letter of the post–1960s generation. Often painful and with no cure, herpes simplex virus 2 was the new poster child for the diseases that just kept on giving. Little did that generation know what was about to erupt—a new disease that was to become a global scourge and redefine sexual behavior for the decades that followed.

If you like a good detective story, the arrival of HIV/AIDS on the American scene is a fascinating tale. In 1981, young men on the West Coast were being afflicted with a deadly type of pneumonia rarely seen before in their age group. The single common factor shared by these men was their homosexuality. At the same time, three thousand miles away on the East Coast, men were also dying from complications of the same type of pneumonia, and their only common connection was intravenous drug abuse—to be specific, sharing needles. Then, a third group of men appeared with a similar sickness, in this case their common bond was a Haitian heritage. Finally, a fourth group of individuals arrived on the scene with the deadly illness; these were hemophiliacs, people who lacked a clotting factor in their blood and required transfusions of blood products.

The epidemiological detectives at the Centers for Disease Control and Prevention (CDC) in Atlanta were finally able to join together pieces of the puzzle to create a more comprehensible picture. Initially calling the disease "gay related" only added to the homophobic atmosphere of the time and provided straight folks with a dangerously false sense of security.

At the outset of the epidemic, heterosexuals accounted for about 1 percent of all infections compared with today's rate of nearly 15 percent. Because of the development of drug treatments in the mid 1990s that seem fairly successful at controlling the replication of the virus for some individuals, many people mistakenly think that AIDS has now been cured and they don't need to worry about it.

Nothing could be further from the truth. I hate to be a downer here, but there is no cure for AIDS, nor do I honestly think there will be one in our lifetime. We have no idea if the medications that seem so successful today will continue to be effective over time, and some people are unable to tolerate some of the harsher side effects of the drugs. AIDS is here to stay, folks, and it's time for everyone to get their heads around the fact that it's a very real issue that we will have to consider for the foreseeable future.

What's the difference between HIV and AIDS?

Human Immunodeficiency Virus (HIV) is the virus believed to cause AIDS (Acquired Immunodeficiency Syndrome). The virus destroys a specific type of white blood cell that would ordinarily protect the body against infections and illness. These infections are called "opportunistic" because they take advantage of the immune system's weakened state to invade the body. Once a person develops one of these infections or illnesses, he or she has progressed from being HIV positive to being a person with AIDS.

Is AIDS no longer a gay disease?

What time warp have you been living in? Although male-to-male transmission was the most common route of infection in the first decade of the epidemic, intravenous drug abuse and heterosexual sex have caught up, and fewer than 50 percent of new AIDS cases each year result from male-to-male sex.

Wasn't the high number of AIDS cases found in the homosexual population due to the fact that that type of sex is just plain wrong and immoral?

Who are you . . . Pat Robertson's long-lost illegitimate child? Let me say this: if AIDS is God's revenge on homosexuals for their bad behavior, then lesbians must be God's chosen people, because they hardly ever get AIDS! And for your information, if anal sex is a major risk factor, then several surveys suggest that around 25 percent of straight couples practice anal sex. Just not you, right?

Is it really true that lesbians don't get AIDS?

There are some known cases of lesbians contracting HIV, but these individuals also had other risk factors like intravenous drug use or blood transfusions, making identification of the cause of the infection impossible. There's always some risk through sexual contact, but the virtual absence of HIV in lesbians without other identified risk factors is dramatic. Someone's looking out for lesbians!

Does anal sex cause AIDS?

A couple of years ago I was teaching the AIDS unit when a young woman at the back of the classroom raised her hand. Her question was, "Does anal sex cause AIDS?" I was about to give her my very erudite response when, before I could speak, she added, "Because my boyfriend wants to put it up my butt, and I'm not sure I should let him!"

After picking myself up off the floor and quieting the howls of delight from her bemused classmates, I informed her that the very act of anal sex cannot *cause* an HIV infection unless the guy on the business end of the penis actually has the infection at the time of rear entry.

Which sexual behaviors are the highest risk for passing on HIV?

The order of risk for HIV transmission would be anal sex, vaginal sex, and oral sex. I think that's it; did I miss an orifice? Kissing is an extremely unlikely risk factor given the much-diluted volume of virus in saliva.

Why is anal sex the highest sexual risk? Is it because it's so freaky?

Says who? There you go again with that judgmental attitude. Disease transmission is about the physiology, not the morality. The vagina is a more "rugged" organ than the anus and lubricates during sexual arousal. The tissues of the anus and rectum do not lubricate naturally and are more prone to microscopic tearing than the vagina, thereby providing easier access to the circulatory system for the invading virus. The virus doesn't care whether it's gaining entry through a vagina or an anus—it's just looking for a home. And remember, a lot of straight folks report having done this "taboo" act!

Can I get infected with HIV by sharing a swimming pool or hot tub?

No chance. Most of the body fluids that would normally get washed off in a pool or tub, like sweat or saliva, are not fluids that would normally transmit HIV. In addition, the volume of water would greatly dilute any virus, to say nothing of the deadly effects of chlorine. Now, if you're having incredible, aquatic sex in the pool or tub, then that's a different matter altogether.

Can I get HIV from someone performing oral sex on me?

If the person providing you the oral service is HIV-positive and a small amount of blood from his or her mouth enters the urethra or vagina, infection is possible. The risk is certainly less than that of anal or vaginal sex, but the risk still exists.

Can I get HIV from performing oral sex on another person?

Although it's not that common, there are some reported cases of the "performer" contracting HIV.

One older diabetic male, who was unable to gain a sufficient erection to have intercourse with his wife, had been secretly visiting a prostitute on the side and performing cunnilingus on her. He contracted HIV and the cunnilingus was his only risk factor—should have stayed home and given his wife some cunnilingus.

Can you get HIV from someone who doesn't have any symptoms?

Absolutely. My guess would be the vast majority of people who have contracted HIV through sexual contact got it from someone who had no symptoms. The incubation period for HIV can be anywhere from six months to more than ten years, during which time the infected person looks absolutely fine. You can't tell by looking—put the condom on!

Can HIV be transmitted from other animals to humans?

No. HIV is a uniquely human disease and the chimpanzee is about the only animal that has developed antibodies to HIV.

Can you get HIV from kissing?

The virus has been identified in saliva but in dilute proportions. It would certainly require huge gobs of saliva over a prolonged period for this activity to transmit HIV, and even then the risk is negligible. And if you're dating someone who's drooling into your mouth when you kiss, you might need to get yourself a new partner.

How soon after sex should I get an HIV test?

Most of the available HIV tests search for an antibody to the virus. The body takes anywhere from three to six months to develop the antibodies. (I don't want to make this a microbiology lesson, but just in case: an antibody is a protein produced by the body's immune system that recognizes and helps fight infection.) So the standard advice would be, get tested three months after your time of risk, and if the result is negative, get retested after another three months. If you're negative after six months have elapsed you can be pretty confident you don't have HIV. The kicker here, though, is you can't have sex without a condom during this six-month period, or the clock will have to be reset.

Where can I get tested and will the testing be anonymous?

Most local county or city health departments offer anonymous HIV testing. You'll simply be given a number to match to a test result. Other sites might require your personal information (name and address) but will keep that data confidential. If your local health department does not offer testing, they should be able to provide a list of local resources. The Centers for Disease Control (CDC) also provides an Internet site called National HIV Testing Resources that will enable an individual to search for a testing site in their area. The Internet address is: www.hivtest.org

What type of tests are there for HIV?

Although some facilities might use a test that examines antigens (foreign substances that when introduced to the body stimulate the production of antibodies) of HIV, most of the available tests look for the presence of antibodies your body might produce in reaction to the virus. The most common type of test has historically been a blood test. However, many facilities today are using a swab to collect a sample of oral mucosa from inside the cheek to test for antibodies.

Will I have to wait long for the test results?

Until 2002, you'd have had to wait several days before you could obtain test results, and many facilities required that you return in person to get them. Such a system was obviously nerve-wracking for the individual awaiting the result, and many individuals were simply too scared to return at all, so they didn't. Some facilities now use a rapid HIV test that usually produces results in up to twenty minutes, so you can be tested and receive a result all in the same day.

Who really needs to get a test for HIV?

I could be politically correct and say everyone, but obviously some people are at much higher risk for infection than others. Over the years I've had students from both ends of a risk continuum. "Dr. Sawyer, I had sex with a girl once, three years ago. Well, it wasn't real sex, I just put my penis against her vagina. I didn't really put it in, but now I'm worried about AIDS. I haven't had sex with anyone since—you think I should get tested?"

Are you kidding me? I've also talked to men at a university STI clinic who'd had multiple sexual partners, never used a condom, and had just been diagnosed with gonorrhea, but when I asked them what they felt their risk was for HIV, they all pretty much said, "zero!" If I'd had a stupid-stick handy I'd have wacked them on the ends of their offending members, but such is the power of denial.

I believe that unless you're in a totally monogamous relationship, if you've had unprotected vaginal or anal intercourse you should get yourself tested for HIV, and if you've given or received oral sex and the worry about HIV is freaking you out, you should also get tested.

Come on . . . do straight men really need to worry about HIV/AIDS? Wouldn't you have to be some type of man-whore to get infected?

Let's examine the numbers. In the early days of AIDS, heterosexual contact accounted for less than 1 percent of AIDS cases. Now that figure is 15 percent. In addition, one of the fastest growing groups with new HIV infection is heterosexual women, and that's where you come in. You tend to hook up with heterosexual women, and given that infected women will pretty much have no symptoms for HIV, good luck with that. Do you realistically have a much greater chance of getting genital warts, chlamydia, gonorrhea, or herpes than HIV? Certainly, but you're still at risk, so why not always use a condom to protect yourself from all these goodies? I know, with this book I've put you off having sex—well, for at least fifteen minutes and three beers, so don't forget the condom.

What's my risk for HIV/AIDS if I've only had a couple of sexual partners?

There's no question, if you reduce your number of different sexual partners, you'll reduce the likelihood of getting HIV, but even a single unprotected act of intercourse puts you at risk, because technically you're not just having sex with that one person. You're now linked to a network of sexual activity that might include more than three hundred individuals.

For example: Chad unexpectedly gets diagnosed with HIV and he's utterly shocked. How did this happen to him? He's a red-blooded, all-American guy, who's never used intravenous (IV) drugs, never had same-gender sex, and never had a blood transfusion (all the traditional high-risk factors). Well, maybe Chad had sex with a girl, who'd had sex with a guy, who'd had sex with a girl, who'd had sex with a guy, who'd had sex with a girl, who'd shot IV drugs . . . and we're not even including the other sexual partners each of these people undoubtedly had, and their partners, and so on and so on. The common phrase, "when you have sex with one person you're having sex with all the people they've had sex with," is absolutely true. When you get over the stunning visual of all those people in one massive bed having sex, you get the point: reducing your number of sexual partners reduces your odds of getting an STI, including HIV, but the risk is still there.

Gay, Bi, or Hopelessly Confused: Alternate Sexual Expression

Here's a newsflash: not everyone you know is heterosexual. Although homosexuality and bisexuality are discussed more openly these days, and contemporary television shows seem to intimate that every hip person should accessorize with a witty, gay sidekick, many people are still pretty ignorant about the whole issue of sexual expression. In an academic sense, very little research has been performed on sexual orientation. In the 1800s, when sexuality research in general started to develop, social scientists were hesitant to examine homosexuality for fear that they would be dubbed as pathological by association. In fact, during this early examination of the issue, some scientists believed that homosexuals were in fact a third gender; you had men, women, and homosexuals.

At the end of the nineteenth century the academic establishment was shocked when researcher Henry Havelock Ellis reported that same-gender sexual behavior existed in every culture. But that was nothing compared to the outcry when Alfred Kinsey rocked everyone's world in the late 1940s with his discourse on American sexual behavior, particularly his scale of sexual orientation.

Kinsey did not believe in discrete categories of sexual orientation, but rather that orientation existed on a continuum from 0–6, with 0 representing total heterosexuality in both psychological fantasy and behavior, and 6 representing a similar position at the homosexual end of the continuum. Points in between 0 and 6 described varying degrees of heterosexual-homosexual orientation.

Kinsey was accused of ruining the fabric of American society. A congressional subcommittee examined the possible disastrous effects of his work on the American family, and the *New York Times* refused to publish a book review on Kinsey's academic tomes. Of course, Kinsey didn't help his case by being, shall we say, a little too physically involved in experiencing some of the fruits of his own research, including same-gender action, but nevertheless his contribution to the understanding of homosexuality was invaluable.

Much has happened in the world of homosexuality

since Kinsey and Havelock Ellis shook the foundations of American culture. The AIDS epidemic exploding in the early eighties further marginalized gays from mainstream culture as they were seen as carriers of the new plague. However, the presence of gay characters on television has become much more commonplace since Billy Crystal played one in a seventies comedy called *Soap*, although many of the more recent characters seem to represent the very effeminate end of the gay male continuum. The opening years of the new millennium have seen the struggle shift to the domain of civil ceremonies and marriage. Vermont became the first state to recognize civil ceremonies for gay couples, Massachusetts the first state to recognize marriage, and that bastion of liberalism, the Netherlands, became the first nation to allow marriage between gay couples.

Since 2004, conservatives in the United States have moved to block same-gender marriage under the smoke screen that it devalues and threatens the sanctity of heterosexual marriage. Since heterosexuals think that marriage is so sacred we feel a need to do it over and over again! How sacred is marriage to heterosexuals? The divorce rate is around 60 percent. Here's my take on this. Within the next twenty years most states will have legalized gay marriage or at least civil unions, and everyone will wonder what the big deal was back in "the day"! In my mind, homosexuals have every right to be just as happy or miserable as the rest of us. Welcome to the club, is what I say.

Does anyone know what causes someone to be gay?

Not really. Anyone who tells you they know for sure is full of it. There are three basic theories: genetics, environment, and a combination of genetics and environment. This is basically the old "nurture versus nature" argument that we've seen played out with other concepts, such as intelligence. The genetics argument suggests that we are born a certain way—straight, gay, or something in between—and there's not much we can do about it. The environmental proponents would describe individuals being born "blank" with sexual orientation determined by upbringing and home environment. The combination argument suggests that individuals are born with a predisposition to being gay or straight but that environment could influence a final outcome.

Are humans the only species to have same-gender sexual contact?

Are you kidding? There are at least five hundred species of animals that have been documented as being involved in same-gender sexual contact. The bonobo, an African ape, is believed to be essentially bisexual, and studies suggest that 75 percent of all sex experienced by these apes is thought to be non-reproductive. They do it for fun, and they do it with the same sex frequently!

Experts have known for a long time that monkeys and great apes have dabbled in same-sex behavior, but we now know that many other species also participate. Male penguin couples have been known to maintain the same partner for life; American bison bulls have been recorded mounting other bulls with full anal penetration; and many bighorn rams spend a great deal of time getting close to another ram's big horns, so to speak.

Is there any difference between sexual orientation and sexual preference?

The term sexual preference suggests to me the concept of choice. That is, I prefer to be gay or straight. Personally, I'm a strong believer in the genetic school of "reason for being gay," so I don't believe that people choose their sexual orientation and I consequently don't like the term "preference." Think about it. Would anyone really choose to be gay in a culture that remains relatively homophobic? "If I choose to be gay, I'll be kicked out of my house, my parents might disown me, I might lose my job, and pretty much lots of people might hate me or even beat me up . . . yeah, that's the ticket, I'll be gay!" That just doesn't make any sense to me. Does any heterosexual ever remember waking up one morning, deciding to be straight? Sounds unlikely.

Is 10 percent of the population really gay?

The 10-percent statistic has been thrown about for years and had its roots in Kinsey's work back in the late forties. However, Kinsey's work was misinterpreted as he never suggested that 10 percent of the U.S. population was gay. Rather, he reported that 4 percent of men and 2 percent of women were exclusively gay (a 6 on his scale). Subsequent studies in the U.S. and Europe have since confirmed Kinsey's estimate. Does it really matter what the actual percentage is? Probably only to certain politicians who are painfully reminded that homosexuals do actually have the vote!

Is it fair to let gay people have or raise kids? Won't they raise them to be gay too?

Let's think about this logically. What was the sexual orientation of the vast majority of parents of gay people? Yes, that would be heterosexual. They raised their children in a heterosexual manner, in a heterosexual home, to live in a predominantly heterosexual world, and yet their children were gay anyway. Therefore, why would it be likely that two homosexual parents would be any more successful at raising a child to be gay? And why should it matter?

*I had lots of boyfriends in high school, but then
I had sex with another woman in my freshman
year of college. Does that mean I'm a lesbian?*

I don't know, but I think it's important that you understand the distinction between behavior and orientation. The unspoken truth about college sexuality
is that experimenting with the same gender is not
that uncommon, but obviously no one talks about it.
"How was your weekend, Scott?" "It was OK. I had
sex with Frank last night. Didn't do much for me, so I
guess I'll just hang with girls all the time!" My feeling
is that if you've always been attracted to men, and
you try sex with a woman once, that doesn't make
you a lesbian. Now, if you keep going back for more
of that good stuff, then we might come to a different conclusion. We also have to consider the possibility of bisexuality. As explained earlier, Alfred Kinsey
supported the idea of a sexual continuum where
absolutes—that is, completely straight or completely
gay—aren't necessarily the norm.

*Some people feel that most bisexuals are really
gay but are reluctant to come out. What's your
take?*

I think if you buy into Kinsey's notion that sexual orientation exists on a continuum, rather than an either/or
model, then I think you have to accept that bisexuality does exist and is not just a cop-out category for

people who are really gay. I don't think it's logical to assume that there are only two possible variations in sexual orientation—homosexual or heterosexual. I think it makes more sense that people who are exclusively gay or straight represent opposite ends of a continuum, with variations in between that include bisexuality. I also think there are variations within bisexuality, where some bisexuals tend to be more same-gender sexually oriented and some opposite-gender sexually oriented.

What about gay sex and that male prison thing?

Being in a same-sex prison for a long period of time offers an interesting situation. What are your sexual choices?

(a) total abstinence,
(b) huge amounts of masturbation,
(c) hooking up with another guy because any human comfort and physical companionship is better than none.

Let's suppose you're a married man but serving a five-year stretch drives you to seek out male companionship. You're released after serving your time and return to your wife. Are you gay now? Many of my students will respond, "Damn right you're gay. Why else would you do that?" I don't necessarily agree. Sounds more like a situational response, one that disappears once the environment changes. But again, if the ex-prisoner continues to dabble in the same-gender stuff, then maybe we'd have to reassess.

If you're a *Sopranos* fan, you might remember Tony's conversation with his therapist where he explains that although homosexuality is totally forbidden within the mafia culture, if a mobster is in prison he's allowed to dabble. He gets a "free pass." Well, if it's OK for the mob, it should be OK for all of us!

My fiancée just admitted to me that she had a same-gender sexual experience about a year before we hooked up. Should I be concerned that she's a lesbian and we shouldn't get married?

Over the years, I've talked about this issue with my students and the responses have been interesting, if somewhat predictable. When a woman shares this information with a man, most of the male responses have been surprise with a tinge of excitement, accompanied by (from the alpha males), "Could you bring a friend over," or "Could I watch?" Men had much less concern than women that sexual orientation might be an issue. If a man told a woman that he'd had a same-sex experience the woman tended to be much less excited about it and very anxious that the male might not be heterosexual. Again, communication and honesty would be paramount in answering this question, although under certain circumstances the individual might not be sure about his or her orientation, but that too should be communicated.

Transvestites are pretty much all gay, aren't they?

Actually, they are pretty much all straight. The majority of transvestites, who are technically labeled with the diagnosis of "transvestic fetishism," are heterosexual men. Because the ridiculous generalization exists that all gay men are effeminate, by slipping into a sexy, slinky dress, surely a man is reinforcing that estrogen-laden persona? Many transvestites cross dress only occasionally and in private, then become sexually aroused and masturbate. Others cross dress more frequently and sometimes join other men in a kind of "show and tell" at a regular gathering. The range of different transvestic behaviors is quite broad, but the sexual orientation of the males involved is not—most are pretty straight!

Does anyone really have "gaydar"? Does it work?

Gaydar . . . the idea that some people have a sixth sense that enables them to scan a crowd and detect a gay person among a mass of heteros, is pretty unlikely. (Sure, if someone's wearing a T-shirt with the logo Queer Nation in giant letters, I guess that's a clue but you hardly need advanced psychic powers to work that out!) Many of the stereotypes of effeminate men and masculinized women come into play here, but often appearances can be deceiving and certainly the vast majority of gay folks simply don't fit these gender-based stereotypes. Traditionally there have been "signs" that some would argue give clues to sexual orientation, like earrings in a left or right ear or a bandanna in a specific back pocket, or even French kissing another guy in a gay bar, but failing the presence of such markers, it's a crapshoot. Gay or straight, we've all made incorrect assumptions about someone's sexual orientation, so the likelihood of "gaydar" or even "straightdar" as a meaningful idea is unlikely.

How come gays are so into anal sex?

Actually, just because a guy is getting it on with another man (who's obviously absent a vagina) doesn't automatically make either of the males aficionados of the nether region. Many gay men do not participate in anal sex and prefer other methods of stimulation like oral sex and/or mutual masturbation. You could also ask why seemingly increased numbers of heterosexual men have developed a liking for the alternative port of entry in their female lovers (see page 112). It's all a question of taste, and every person has his or her own sexual repertoire that gets played out, regardless of sexual orientation—gay or straight doesn't necessarily define specific sexual activity.

I Seem to Have a Little Problem: Sexual Dysfunction

Sexual dysfunction . . . quite simply, a psycho-babble term for when things go wrong sexually. Until very recently, public discussion of sexual difficulty was considered taboo. Women's sexual problems were all but ignored and any man foolish enough to go public with a problem was immediately viewed as suspect, and possibly pathological. We've seen an amazing turnaround in the level of advertising, particularly televised commercials, for products to alleviate the problem of erectile dysfunction (ED). Such a quick switch caught the American public napping, and before they knew what was happening, men watching their Sunday afternoon football games were asked by their inquisitive middle schoolers why that older couple was lying in adjacent baths on the top of a mountain, waiting for the right moment to arise—whatever that might mean. One minute it's all football, Chevy trucks, and Miller Lite, and the next it's "Can you still get it up, Dad?" Amazing.

Our stereotypes of who is likely to experience sexual dysfunction is colored by antiquated ideas and usually involves descriptors like "old," "male," and we may as well throw in "dirty" just to round things out. Although older individuals are indeed more likely to experience sexual dysfunction, plenty of younger people have difficulties with sex, including premature ejaculation, inorgasmia, and erectile dysfunction. My take on this whole issue is no matter what your age, if you're sexually active, at some point you're almost bound to suffer from a sexual dysfunction.

Take the example of one of my students a few years ago. He was a good-looking, twenty-one-year-old senior who was due to graduate that semester, and he had a serious problem. With his *GQ* looks and a quick wit, he had no difficulty attracting some hot women. But despite being able to make out with an erection, or successfully masturbate to ejaculation, as soon as he attempted vaginal penetration, he would lose his erection. This nightmare had continued unabated for almost his entire four years of college, and he had told no one. How would you? "Had a good weekend, Bill?" "No, not really, I couldn't get it up again!"

I told him that if he could find a partner with whom

he could develop a solid relationship before having intercourse, maybe she could help him work through the difficulty. He responded the problem was that when he went out with women they usually wanted to have sex almost immediately (and that's a problem, you say? I can hear the groans of envy from here!), so rather than going through the humiliation of an almost inevitable embarrassing failure, the student had completely stopped dating and basically become a social recluse. I referred the student to a sex therapist in the community. I repeat, he was young, good-looking, and in no way dirty—get the message? Dysfunction can happen to anyone.

A female student approached me with great embarrassment to explain that she was freaking out because her twenty-year-old boyfriend took forever to ejaculate—on most occasions, nearly an hour. (Again, I can hear the partners of premature ejaculators screaming, "I could use some of that action!") Maybe you could, but you know, people have things to do, places to be, and they can't always be waiting for Vesuvius to erupt once every damn Ice Age. As a woman, my student had been well socialized to believe that:

(a) she must be doing something wrong,
(b) she was useless in bed,
(c) she wasn't sexy enough,
(d) her boyfriend didn't really like her anymore.

Given how women have been conditioned to feel responsible for almost all relationship issues, my student's feelings were understandable, but totally incorrect. Boyfriend needed some big help with his problem—delayed ejaculation. It was off to the sex therapist with this nice, clean young man. I think you're getting the point.

What's the most common sexual dysfunction in men?

The most common sexual dysfunction in men, young men in particular, is premature ejaculation or "coming too soon." The difficulty with this dysfunction is defining exactly what it is. For example, can you place a minimum time limit on ejaculation? If Jake usually ejaculates in three minutes (it was a good night) but is dating a partner who orgasms in two minutes, is Jake a premature ejaculator? Probably not, but only as long as he doesn't change partners. If Jake gets dumped and his new partner takes about five minutes to orgasm, now poor old Jake has got himself a big problem.

Believe it or not, one university study tried to define premature ejaculation by pelvic thrust quotients. The same premise that applied to timing Jake's ejaculation applies to the number of thrusts—it's all relative. I like to define premature ejaculation as simply the inability to control when you ejaculate, but here comes the all-important caveat—*within reason*. Don't believe what you see in those oh-so realistic porn films where the actor is banging away for what seems like an eternity. (Not that the average porn viewer watches more than three minutes of the movie anyway, but you see my point.) For starters, haven't you ever heard of film editing, and second, those guys are professionals, for goodness sake; they're not like the rest of us, who have day jobs and don't have time to be hitting it like that for hours on end.

How is premature ejaculation treated?

Here comes the good news. The typical treatment for premature ejaculation usually involves practicing—masturbation and intercourse, that is. Think of ejaculation as a cliff edge, and you don't want to fall over too soon. You would masturbate until you're close to the cliff edge, then stop. This activity would be repeated over time until some control is established. Then perhaps a partner will masturbate you and this will necessitate your communicating with your partner as the cliff edge looms—screaming "stop!" usually suffices. Then you might penetrate your partner and again establish the cliff edge ("don't move, oh please, God, don't move") until you develop some control.

Of course, as every man will testify, he will eventually arrive at a point of no return (ejaculatory inevitability as we say, in the biz), where he can no longer hold back his ejaculation. That will be the time to let it go, plunging blissfully over the cliff edge.

Masters and Johnson developed a rather more

"vigorous" treatment in the 1960s called the "squeeze technique" that, simply stated, comprises the male taking the base or tip of his penis between forefinger and thumb and squeezing like hell immediately prior to ejaculation. Does that prevent ejaculation? Oh yes, it usually gets the job done, but unless a little pain is your thing, I think most men prefer the stop-start method described above.

Are there things men can do to last longer?

Most people have swapped tactics about this issue (usually in their teen years) and a couple of universals seem to exist: think about something else, like baseball, soccer, vegetables, your grandmother, absolutely anything but what's going on at that moment. And do you know what? That's completely the opposite of what actually works—what a shocker! Premature ejaculation is treated by masturbation in conjunction with a focus on sensations, where the individual is encouraged to concentrate precisely on what he is feeling, how close he is to ejaculating and extending the metaphor, the location of the orgasmic cliff edge. By thinking of something else and not concentrating on sensations, the man is absolutely giving up control.

Another recommendation often heard echoing through high school hallways is for males to masturbate prior to subsequent intercourse. There is, in fact, a grain of truth to this idea in that if you haven't ejaculated for weeks or even months before having sex, you are certainly less likely to last very long compared to the individual who has recently been active. However, this method isn't that dependable and most typical premature ejaculators are still likely to have problems with their timing.

What's the most common sexual dysfunction in younger women?

The most common sexual dysfunction in younger women is female orgasmic disorder, also known as inorgasmia or anorgasmia—the inability to achieve an orgasm. However, remember that men and women differ here. Although most men would howl at the prospect of sexual intercourse without orgasm, a heterosexual woman who can consistently climax through penis-vagina intercourse alone is in the minority.

What percentage of women are unable to have an orgasm?

This isn't an easy question to answer. Do you mean orgasm *every time* women have intercourse? Does masturbation count? You see the problem. Some recent studies would suggest that approximately 10 percent of sexually active women never have orgasms through any sexual activity and an additional 10–15 percent rarely experience them.

What are some of the reasons for inorgasmia?

Some of the leading reasons for inorgasmia (inability to orgasm) in women include lack of foreplay, fatigue, preoccupation with nonsexual thoughts, and partner ejaculating too soon after penetration. Are you paying attention, men? One factor that seems to unite many women who experience inorgasmia is lack of experience with self-touch or masturbation. Unlike males, who are inevitably ecstatic about having to masturbate to reduce the likelihood of prostate cancer, some women are less than comfortable touching themselves sexually, even though this is for purely medicinal purposes.

Do you think not being able to have an orgasm might be genetic?

Sounds weird, but genes might actually play a role. A 2007 study on twin females performed at St. Thomas's Hospital in London reported that one-third of the women never or hardly ever experienced orgasms, and researchers suggested that as much as 60 percent of this sexual dysfunction could be accounted for by genetics. I doubt the following will be of much comfort to inorgasmic women, but a theory put forward by the researchers was that maybe, far from being a defect, the failure of some women to orgasm is actually a refined mate-selection tool, the idea being that only men skilled in the art of love-

DR ROBIN SAWYER

making and who care about the woman's satisfaction will be able to help her orgasm, and thus be a good choice to stick around as a long-term mate. So according to this theory, women who orgasm too easily are the ones with the problem. It's just a wild shot in the dark, but given the choice between an evolutionary mate-selection tool that provides a climax once a decade, and lashings of easy orgasms on a daily basis, I think most women would take their chances with men of inferior quality!

If a woman is unable to orgasm through penis-vagina sex, should she consider this a sexual dysfunction?

It depends. Are we talking every time she has sex, or sporadically? Clearly, most individuals would agree that if a heterosexual woman never has an orgasm through penis-vagina sex, then that's probably a dysfunction. However, many experts believe that if the lack of orgasm isn't perceived as a "problem" by a particular woman, then technically it should not be considered a dysfunction. Putting aside the incredulity of some women and definitely all men who will be asking, "Are you kidding? Never have an orgasm and that's not a problem?" a school of thought does exist suggesting that the individual's *perception* is more important than an external diagnosis. This goes back to something we discussed earlier, the "I don't orgasm but the foreplay's great" phenomenon. Some women may be reconciled to not experiencing orgasm and gain pleasure from the sexual activity that would usually precede climax. So you can see, this issue isn't quite as clear as it might appear at first glance because there's a huge *it depends* attached.

My girlfriend swears she doesn't mind not having an orgasm every time we have sex. Do you think she really means that or is she just being a martyr?

I think she's getting it somewhere else from a battery-powered device or a stud who knows what he's doing in bed and she's just humoring you to save your feelings. Is that what you want to hear? I know this is revolutionary news for men, but you have to start embracing the fact that most men and women have different patterns of sexual response.

In the recent National Health and Social Life Survey only 29 percent of women reported "always" having an orgasm with their partners during the past year. By contrast, 41 percent of the women said they were "extremely physically satisfied by sex," and 39 percent reported feeling "extreme emotional satisfaction" with their partners. In other words, for many women, having an orgasm is not tied to being physically and emotionally satisfied with sex.

Here comes the kicker: although 75 percent of men reported "always" having an orgasm during

D
R

R
O
B
I
N

S
A
W
Y
E
R

sex, their reported emotional and physical satisfaction rates were only 47 percent and 42 percent respectively. Although men were more than twice as likely to achieve an orgasm every time they had sex, the men were barely more likely than the women to report being emotionally or physically satisfied with sex. So, interestingly, orgasm isn't exactly a great predictor of sexual satisfaction for men either.

What's the treatment for female orgasmic disorder?

Most treatments combine various approaches that might include communication skills training, cognitive restructuring, sex education, therapy, and perhaps the most well documented treatment, masturbation. Masturbation is often recommended as a means of encouraging a woman to become more comfortable with her body and sexual response. Although learning to masturbate to orgasm has been one of the most successful treatments to date, some therapists refrain from using it, often because of an individual's discomfort with the practice.

When I masturbate or use a vibrator, the orgasms I experience seem so much more intense than when I have sex with my boyfriend. I feel bad about this and don't feel I can tell him. How can I achieve the same level of satisfaction with him?

Oh no, man has been replaced by a AAA battery vibrator and destined to always be second best! Not to worry, what you're describing is nothing new. Back in the sixties, Masters and Johnson reported that women were most likely to experience a more intense orgasm through masturbation than through penis-vagina sex. It's okay, as most guys don't really care how intense your big O is anyway; they're too concerned about their own. But why not try this: incorporate your vibrator or whatever toy you prefer in your solo sex play into your sex play with the guy and maybe you'll have sex that'll curl your toes. And the Energizer Bunny just keeps on goin'.

After losing my virginity, how long before I'm comfortable in bed and able to orgasm?

This theme of discomfort among women, and inability to feel much of anything, never mind an orgasm, is sadly so frequent, it's almost the norm. Unlike the hyped up, intimate, romantic Hollywood version of virginity loss, where the boy lasts for hours and hours and the girl experiences mind-rocking multiple orgasms, the reality of neophyte sex is very different.

In one of my research studies I asked students to reflect back on their loss of virginity experience and score their physical satisfaction, from 1 (awful) to 10 (fantastic). The male mean was a surprisingly mediocre 5, while the female mean was a pathetic 2. Hardly equates to the Hollywood version, does it?

When asked how many of the students reached an orgasm during first-time intercourse, the results were also interesting. Ninety-two percent of men achieved an orgasm (I have no idea what the other 8 percent were doing), while only 6 percent of women climaxed. What's become evident to me is that it takes much longer for women to become comfortable with their sexuality, and that for many young women in particular, sexual intercourse often provides little pleasure at first. The good news is that most women do become more comfortable over time, particularly if they can find a caring partner, rather than just one who is looking for someone to get him off.

Do young men really experience erectile dysfunction or is that just a story made up by old guys to make them feel better about their problem?

Although the majority of erectile dysfunction sufferers do tend to be older men, several studies have shown that relatively high proportions of young men are also experiencing a problem getting it up. Dr. Irwin

Goldstein, a renowned urologist from Boston specializing in sexual response, estimates the prevalence of erectile dysfunction (ED) among college-aged men to be approaching 25 percent. Unfortunately, devastated by their untimely affliction, many of these men feel too embarrassed to seek medical help, and their problem goes unresolved. If you have a "friend" who has a problem with ED, tell him to get some help. He could talk to his general practitioner or a urologist. Look at the numbers; he's clearly not alone.

Are some younger males using Viagra recreationally?

Viagra is intended for use by men who have problems with ED and works by relaxing smooth muscle, resulting in vasodilation and increased blood flow to the penis and, ultimately, a more effective erection. However, Viagra has become popular on the urban club scene, where the drug is amusingly called "Poke"—you've got to love that name.

Poke is often used in conjunction with other recreational drugs like Ecstasy to provide the user with a terrific chance of experiencing a heart attack—what a way to go! Again, Viagra is designed to help men overcome ED, not to provide superfluous perpetual erections for the party crowd—and a potentially dangerous erection at that.

Did I hear there was an injection you could have to get an erection?

Yes. An injection of a drug called Papaverine can produce a chemically induced erection, but I should mention that the medication is injected directly into the penis. Still want it? Long before the little blue pill called Viagra made getting an erection a piece of cake, some men were using the aforementioned injection to achieve the same thing. Next came a pellet called alprostadil which men inserted into the end of their penises. Would that be better or worse than the needle? Let's take a moment to honor pioneers who truly paid a high price for maintaining their sex lives. Anyone can take a pill.

What are the possible causes of a guy not ejaculating during sex with a girl he is comfortable with and finds attractive?

If this is more than an occasional problem, the male in question could have what is known as inhibited or delayed ejaculation. Some men (and their partners) would pay money for this problem as they're on the opposite end of the ejaculatory spectrum. Men who suffer from inhibited ejaculation are often able to masturbate or receive oral sex to the point of orgasm, but cannot ejaculate during penetrative sex. The most common reasons for this problem are unconscious feelings of anxiety, whatever the cause, and in certain instances, feelings of guilt or conflict. Usually, a male would need to work with a therapist in an attempt to uncover the causes of the psychological conflicts that are affecting his ability to ejaculate.

Sometimes I'm too tired for sex and my boyfriend takes it personally. Do you think there's something wrong with me, and is there some way I can let him know it's nothing to do with him?

So you don't want to have sex every day of the year? What are you, some type of freak? What you are is actually someone who's pretty normal, and believe it or not many women and even some men don't want to have sex 365 days a year. Now, having said that, many men, on the other hand, simply can't relate to a day without sex. To them, turning down an opportunity is simply not a part of their psyche and the only reason these men might go a day or two without sex is the shortage of a warm body.

Traditionally, heterosexual men have been hungry pursuers, never sure where the next sexual meal was coming from, and when a regular supply has been attained, the man is always fearful that at some point the supply will be withdrawn. Hence his need and compulsion to dine constantly, many times when he isn't even that hungry!

You simply need to reassure your mate that he's a lovely guy, his supply will not be withdrawn any time soon, and that you'd be willing to compromise with a quick hand job. Or you could tell him to shut up because you're going to sleep.

My girlfriend sometimes doesn't lubricate very much and so sex can be painful. Is this normal, and what can we do?

Unlike most young men who can become fully erect at the drop of a hat, women's sexual response tends to be more varied. Some women lubricate vaginally very quickly with generous amounts of lubrication, while others take longer to lubricate and seem to produce smaller amounts of fluid. In some cases, lack of lubrication might simply mean that the woman is not sufficiently stimulated. If whatever you consider foreplay takes less than thirty seconds, you might try increasing those activities.

However, if this problem continues, the woman has several options. She could use a water-based lubricant like Astroglide or K-Y; she could try a vaginal moisturizer like Replens or Lubrin; or if the lack of lubrication is thought to be because of reduced levels of estrogen, the woman could try vaginal estrogen therapy, which could be a cream, a vaginal ring, or pills. Lubricants should be viewed as providing short-term help to reduce levels of discomfort during intercourse. Moisturizers help to replenish the moisture levels of the vagina, working to correct an underlying problem, and can be effective for up to three days.

Although lack of lubrication is traditionally associated with postmenopausal women, a recent study reported that as many as 20 percent of sexually active women have complained of this problem.

This response assumed that your girlfriend is a more than enthusiastic and willing sexual partner. Lack of lubrication can also occur when a woman is consciously or subconsciously conflicted about having sex and vaginal dryness becomes a symptom of this discomfort.

He Wants to Put What Where? Atypical Sexual Behavior

OK, this is the alternative section, the weird stuff that you've been waiting for, you sickos. Now please notice that I didn't title this section *abnormal* sexual behavior, because that would be judgmental, and I wouldn't want anyone to feel badly about their little peccadilloes.

So what are atypical sexual behaviors? Let's just say that although these behaviors aren't practiced by the majority of folks, enough individuals are into them that they have gained recognition. Some atypical sexual behaviors are illegal, some aren't but probably should be, and some are just plain difficult to understand. One of my female students asked in class why men seemed to get off so much on sex from the rear position (see page 111). Before the male students could respond, the woman continued, "I don't mind the rear entry thing but when the guy starts yelling "Yee haw!" and slapping my ass (at which point she illustrated her point by standing and vigorously slapping her buttocks), does he think I'm freakin' Seabiscuit?" I would say different strokes for different folks but that would be gratuitous!

We've already talked about how influential the brain is in human sexuality, and that whole concept really plays out in this section. Think about how many thousands of different ways there are to become sexually stimulated. If you can think of them, then I can guarantee that somewhere in the history of the world, someone has done them. Most of us have differing tastes in all walks of life, and it turns out that sex is no different. Some people believe that certain behaviors are disgusting, horrible, immoral, and possibly should be illegal, while others feel that nothing should be out of bounds for consenting adults and that the limitless range of the human imagination is there to be explored. It's really up to you to decide.

An entire book could be dedicated to human sexual activity that either disgusts or titillates. Here's a brief look at just some of the possibilities.

Is it true that some people actually have sex with animals?

Let's suppose you're dating a guy called Pete, and he seems overly affectionate toward your German shepherd . . . that's zoophilia! Or is it bestiality? Some people use the two terms interchangeably, while others would argue that the terms are not synonymous.

Zoophilia is commonly defined as an affinity or sexual attraction by a human to an animal, while bestiality is considered by some individuals to mean human-animal sexual activity, more of a one-night stand. To make matters more complicated, a new term, "zoosexual," has been developed that describes a broader spectrum of human-animal interaction.

Many men who have sex with animals do so because they live in rural areas where access to "animals" of a two-legged variety might be limited. If this is the case, when those men and women relocate to more populous environs where Fido is not the best bet in town, they tend to revert to more "traditional" sexual outlets, like human beings.

Kinsey reported experience with animals in 8 percent of his male and 4 percent of his female survey respondents. Male contact tends to be with farm animals and involves penile-vagina intercourse, while women are more likely to have contact with household pets and experience the animals licking their genitalia. Perhaps we're becoming more accepting of the practice, as unless it causes a person distress or interferes with normal functioning, zoophilia is no longer classified as a pathology under the American Psychiatric Association's criteria. I wonder what the animals think?

I heard someone talking about "golden showers." What is that?

The technical term for "golden showers" or "water sports" as it is sometimes known, is urophilia. This is where one person urinates on another person who is usually masturbating. To save the carpets, this activity is usually done in the bathtub.

How about coprophilia?

Coprophilia or "scat" is the use of feces to stimulate someone sexually, just like golden showers except this time someone defecates on another person who is masturbating. And you thought someone had "shat" on you at some point in your life? Not like this!

Some guy rubbed up and down against me on the subway last week. Is there a name for that?

I could think of a lot of names for the guy who did that, but the activity is known as "frotteurism" and usually occurs on crowded trains or buses when passengers are packed tightly together. The man rubs his genitals against someone standing in front of him before moving away, and quite often the man's sexual excitement is heightened by the fact that the victim is often unaware of what he's doing, usually due to the densely packed train or bus. Obviously, such physical contact would be considered sexual assault and the perpetrator subject to arrest if he was caught.

My girlfriend flashed her boobs at Mardi Gras last year. I know she was pretty drunk, but do you think she might have a problem?

The activity of exposing one's genitalia is known as exhibitionism, although most people call it flashing, and this activity accounts for as many as one-third of all sex convictions in the U.S., Canada, and Europe. Most true exhibitionists have a compulsive need to expose themselves and are in dire need of help. It's not really a serious pathology, unless you can't stop. Flashing your boobs at Mardi Gras, or that uniquely American phenomenon of "mooning" would probably be considered a harmless prank. Streaking also falls into the mooning category, usually done as a youthful prank at a sporting event and rarely requiring the attention of a therapist.

Is it even possible for women to be true exhibitionists?

Although rare, there are documented cases of exhibitionism in women. Given that a female exhibitionist probably wants to appear sexy and have men admire her body, our culture's social and fashion mores do permit women the opportunity to wear revealing clothing in many situations, so perhaps this exposure may be sufficient to satisfy a female exhibitionist.

What about a guy who's a Peeping Tom? What's that called?

A Peeping Tom, technically a voyeurist, is usually a man who tries to look into bedroom and/or bathroom windows to catch a glimpse of someone undressing, bathing, or even better, having sex. A true voyeurist prefers voyeurism to sexual intimacy with another person.

Why Tom and not Bill or Jack? Legend has it that in the medieval English city of Coventry, the ruler's daughter, Lady Godiva, was so upset about how her father was oppressing the city's people that she made a bargain to ride naked through the streets if her father would promise to reduce taxation. All the citizens of Coventry, out of respect for Lady Godiva, closed their shutters and curtains and no one looked, except one person—a tailor named Tom. Good stuff, this, isn't it? Anyway, voyeurists look into windows, sometimes masturbating while they watch, or perhaps going elsewhere to masturbate while recalling what they have seen. These men are frequently arrested since their sexual excitement tends to increase in response to the likelihood of their getting caught.

What is sadomasochism?

Sadism is named after the infamous eighteenth century French nobleman the Marquis de Sade, who made quite a name for himself writing about the erotic pleasures of inflicting pain. Masochism was named after Leopold von Sacher-Masoch, a nineteenth-century Austrian novelist who expounded on the pleasures of being hurt. So you see, the perfect date is a sadist with a masochist. There'd be no point in two masochists going out together as they'd always be arguing, "Beat me, beat me!" "No, *you* beat *me*!"

The degree of pain inflicted or received can range from the benign, like a "hickey," or to use the English idiom, a "love bite," all the way to a harsh beating, whipping, or cutting with knives or razors. Role-playing is often used to heighten sexual response, particularly in the area of discipline, where elaborate scenarios are sometimes developed to justify the punishment—"who's been a naughty boy, then?" Several high-class prostitutes have reported that they spend more time chasing men around rooms with a whip than they do on their back having sex. It takes all sorts!

Tied up in knots . . . what's the deal with that?

The idea of being tied up is appealing to individuals who like the rush of being controlled and at the total mercy of someone else. This activity, known as bondage, represents the "B" in "B and D"—bondage and discipline. Again, the notion is that someone has been a bad boy, or girl, as, yes, women do get into this too, and for their punishment will be tied up and spanked, whipped, slapped, or whatever else they fancy.

What is klismaphilia?

This is the act of getting a sexual charge from having an enema. For those unfamiliar with the mechanics of this bowel-cleansing procedure, an enema involves the introduction of a liquid solution into the rectum and colon via the anus. To put it a little less clinically, you take a pouch filled with liquid and squirt it through a hose into your ass. Some folks seem to enjoy it.

What is mysophilia?

This is a fun activity for those with sensitive olfactory attributes, aka being a good "sniffer." A mysophiliac is someone who becomes sexually aroused in the presence of underwear that has been worn, stereotypically a male getting his hands on a woman's panties. Often the level of sexual excitement is proportionate to the odor of the panties, so nicely clean, laundered panties may not do the trick. If you've ever lost your panties at the Laundromat *before* you put them in the washing machine, they just might have been lifted by a sniffer!

What is retifism?

This is a shoe fetish, typically a male becoming aroused in the presence of women's shoes. The most likely types of shoes that seem to appeal to the lover of footwear are spiked high heels and knee-length leather boots.

What is scoptophilia?

This activity is similar to voyeurism, but tends to be much more specific; it's getting sexually aroused from secretly observing others having sexual intercourse. This obviously differs from watching porn, as the participants having sex are in the flesh, so to speak, and the scoptophiliac's thrill is derived from the fact that the couple having sex don't know that they're being observed.

What is necrophilia?

Bluntly stated, this is having sex with a dead person. If you consider the physics of the act, it pretty much has to be a male having sex with the corpse. This extremely rare occurrence seems to be the exclusive domain of young men who often get a job in a morgue or funeral home. As you can't exactly get a dead body at your local grocery store, and perhaps can't get a job at a funeral parlor, some men, who would be considered pseudonecrophiliacs, often act out their necrophilic tendencies by having their sexual partners use lots of white face powder to mimic the appearance of death, dress in a funeral shroud, and lie very still during sex. Individuals who practice necrophilia are obviously deeply disturbed and I suppose it would be both superfluous and tasteless to suggest that their having problems with communication would be an understatement.

What's autoerotic asphyxiation (AEA), and is it really dangerous?

D
R

R
O
B
I
N

S
A
W
Y
E
R

Let's put it this way, you have to ask yourself the question, "Is sex worth dying for?" This activity is based on the premise that if you reduce the amount of oxygen reaching the brain as you become sexually aroused, the orgasm you experience will be more intense as you feel a type of hypoxic euphoria. The obvious problem is one of completing your orgasm before passing out and ultimately asphyxiating. This practice hit the headlines in the 1980s when *Hustler* magazine published an article called "Orgasms of Death." In 1987 Larry Flynt, the publisher of the magazine, was taken to court when a fourteen-year-old boy was found hanged with a copy of the magazine at his feet. An initial Texas court found the magazine guilty and responsible for the boy's death but the verdict was later overturned by an appellate court on First Amendment grounds. AEA is most popular in the adolescent male population aged between 13–20 years, and is nothing to play around with—stick with the more mundane orgasm, at least it won't be your last!

Is sexual addiction for real or is that just a bunch of folks who really, really like sex?

Thinks about sex all the time, gets as much sex as he can, watches lots of hot porn, masturbates on a daily basis—sounds like a regular all-American guy, doesn't it? So how do you define a sex addict? Although a "normal" horny male may share some of the same attributes and preoccupations as a sex addict, there are some important differences. Dr. Patrick Carnes, a psychologist and one of the first practitioners to describe this condition in the 1980s, believes that as many as sixteen million men and women are sex addicts. They share some of the same behaviors: compulsive masturbation, use of pornography, chronic sexual affairs, exhibitionism, dangerous sexual practices, prostitution, anonymous sex, compulsive sexual episodes, and voyeurism. More telling still is the list of potential losses/damages experienced by the addict as a result of his or her compulsion: loss of partner or spouse, strained relations with partner, loss of career, unwanted pregnancies, abortions, suicidal thoughts, suicide attempts, and exposure to HIV/AIDS and other sexually transmitted diseases. Sexual addiction shares many of the same compulsive elements as other addictions like alcohol, illicit drugs, and gambling and can be every bit as destructive. As with any serious addiction, treatment involves a great deal of therapy, requires an excellent support system, and to be successful can take a lifetime of commitment.

Is There Sex in My Future?
Sexuality and Aging

A section on aging in a sex book, are you kidding? Every generation thinks that it invented sex, that oral sex wasn't discovered until 1985, and that anyone over the age of thirty-five stopped having sex after their last child was born. Whenever I really want to gross out my students I ask them to think about their parents having sex. The groans, sighs, and gagging sounds are just beginning to clear the air when I hit them with a really low blow. "How about your grandparents?" Sitting around the Thanksgiving table is never quite the same for my students when I've finished with them!

Society has done a marvelous job of selling sex as the domain of hard-bodied, nubile youth, resigning the old-ies to a spirited game of Scrabble, or at best a friendly cuddle. Studies performed in the nineties asking college students about their perceptions of parental sex were met with intense disgust, some students being sufficiently vexed to write on the surveys retorts like, "Who but perverts thinks about their parents having sex?" and "Which dumb-assed person made up this survey?"

The findings of the studies create a world where Mom and Dad obviously did very few sexual things before marriage, with daughters denying any parental premarital sexual contact, and sons grudgingly admitting that the old man must have done some groping around before saying "I do." About one-fourth of the students believed their parents never had intercourse anymore, or not more than a couple of times a year. To make matters worse, when these same students were asked to say whether or not they thought their parents were happily married and still in love, 90 percent of them said "absolutely"! So let me get this right. A married couple that has sex once a year or less is going to be blissfully happy? Even Walt Disney couldn't script that story.

Look, I'm going to do you hard-bodied, beautiful, sexy men and women under the age of thirty-five a huge favor. This will probably be the most exciting section of this book; you just don't know it yet. Here's the reality—unless you experience some tragic accident scuba diving in the Caribbean, or receive a terminal diagnosis as you're ascending Everest, you will get older. Then one day, after you've blinked and it's been two decades since you had insane, mindless, spring-break sex with the Johnson twins in the Fort Lauderdale Super-8 motel, a pimply, barely postpubescent youth will catch you looking a little too closely at a passing twentysomething and shoot you a look of utter disgust. It's officially over—you've creeped out a teenager. You'll want to shout, "Hey, wait a minute, I've still got it. This is me; I'm still the same guy; I really am. Come on, bring out the Johnson twins; no dammit, make it triplets, I can do 'em all!"

Because here's the truth about aging for both men and women—although the years pass and you might become more experienced and hopefully wiser, inside your head you pretty much remain the same person. Despite the passing years, which can include a power job, mortgage, and family, many of us are still waiting to grow up.

Here's the big secret about sex. The single most influential predictor about your sex life as an older person is—you've guessed it—your sex life as a younger person. The truly exciting news is that if you have a healthy attitude and appetite for sex as a young adult, all things being equal with your health, you'll feel the same in middle and older age; your feelings won't change. Isn't that awesome? But, now *you'll* have to learn to live with the same reactions of incredulity mixed with disgust from the younger generations that us "oldies" do now, unless you can start an enlightened social movement to change those ideas, for which the chances are doubtful.

Are you serious that people in their fifties and sixties are having megasex?

Quick sociology lesson. Nearly 78 million Americans were born between 1946 and 1964. These folks represent what we call the baby boomer generation, who, by the way, came of age in the era of sex, drugs, and rock and roll, so they aren't used to sitting around playing checkers. In a country with a divorce rate of over 50 percent, the Census Bureau estimated that 29 percent of adults aged 45–59 were unattached in 2003—that's a lot of singles. Of this group, 70 percent say they date regularly, and 45 percent of men and 38 percent of women have intercourse at least once a week. That's probably more than you get it! Kills you, doesn't it? Folks older than your parents are getting more than you, but the really good news is, that could be you one day.

Is it really OK to be having sex at that age?

As long as you're healthy, there's absolutely no reason why anyone shouldn't have sex into old age. But there is a potential problem. Sixty-one percent of sexually active older singles report having unprotected intercourse. This is a generation that was probably married and therefore insulated against HIV/AIDS and the other sexually transmitted diseases that proliferated during the past twenty years and now has little idea about negotiating safer sex. For example,

D
R

R
O
B
I
N

S
A
W
Y
E
R

from 1990–2004 the number of AIDS cases in adults aged fifty and over increased sevenfold. The potential peril of unprotected sex is one constant you can count on, no matter how old you are.

What's sex like for an old person?

Let's be realistic, your grandpa is probably not doing your grandma doggie style in front of a porn flick after sessions of jaw-numbing oral sex. Unlike younger men and women where sex may take up a much greater proportion of their physical and mental energy, the elderly have lives that are a bit more balanced, and their sexual behavior mirrors that difference. It's not uncommon for an eighty-year-old man to perhaps be unable to ejaculate every time he has intercourse, or for an older woman to experience reduced vaginal lubrication, but from case studies of elderly men and women we begin to see a shift in appreciating sexual and intimate contact for contact's sake, not simply to achieve an orgasm. For a man in particular, that type of concept when he was twenty years younger would have been unthinkable. It's a fact of life—older men and women can still appreciate and participate in the joy of sex. As W. Somerset Maugham so aptly wrote, "Old age has its pleasures, which, though different, are not less than the pleasures of youth."

How about single, elderly people living in group homes. Do they have sex?

Can't you just see it? Mr. Jones wheeling himself down to Room 302 to have a "nooner" with Mrs. Jackson? Given that most men die earlier than women, a healthy, single man in an assisted living environment will be a popular guy. However, some residential settings have an institutional prohibition against such sexual activity, mainly because they don't want to be sued by their residents' adult children, who might be horrified at the prospect of their mother or father still being sexually active. Obviously, families want to be sure that their aging parent is not being abused, but all things being equal, you'd hope the residents are old enough to make their own decisions about a sex life.

Use it or lose it?

If we're talking vaginas here, truer words have never been spoken. Research by Masters and Johnson has clearly shown that regular sexual intercourse or masturbation seems to keep the vagina more elastic and able to lubricate, and helps with maintaining muscle tone and mucus secretions. There's definitely some symmetry here. Masturbating is medically prescribed for young men to reduce their risk of prostate cancer, and intercourse and masturbation is a must for older women to keep their vaginas in healthy shape.

Do women have problems reaching orgasm when they're older?

Although there is some evidence to suggest that women may experience orgasms a little less intensely as they age, this isn't true for all women, and the actual ability to achieve orgasm isn't usually affected by the process of aging. There is no reason why a woman who achieves orgasm as a younger woman won't continue achieving orgasm as an older woman. In fact, some experts believe that women who have completed menopause and are liberated from the worry of unintended pregnancy often find sex to be more enjoyable and satisfying.

Can men still get erections later in life?

Absolutely. When a man gets into his seventies and eighties, his erection might be a little less firm and take longer to achieve, but he should still be able to become erect. Remember now, it takes a younger man all of 5–10 seconds to become erect, so when we say it will take an older man longer, we're not talking an hour here, just a few seconds longer. In addition, the recent development of effective erectile disorder drugs like Viagra and Cialis has enabled many older men to achieve and maintain erections.

Do drugs like Viagra and Cialis really work?

These have been some of the most successful drugs at combating erectile dysfunction. Although these types of drugs don't work for everyone, they do help a large majority of men. A study of Viagra resulted in an overall effectiveness rate of 70 percent, depending on the problem: psychogenic (psychological), 80 percent; prostatectomy (removal of the prostate), 40 percent; diabetes, 55 percent; and spinal cord injury, 60 percent.

How soon after taking one of these drugs do you get an erection?

These drugs don't work that way. Some men mistakenly believe that seconds after taking a little pill, they'll be blessed with a huge, incredibly hard erection, with which you could hammer nails into a wall! All the drugs do is relax smooth muscle to increase blood flow into the penis. You still require sexual stimulation to achieve the erection and your penis isn't just going to leap out of your pants all on its own! Viagra will be effective approximately thirty minutes after taking the pill and can be used up to four hours after consumption. Some men prefer Cialis because this medication can be effective up to thirty-six hours after taking so you can be in less of a hurry.

How about that refractory period thing? Will that be longer?

Yes it will. An older male in his sixties will obviously take longer than a younger man to recover from intercourse and be able to have sex again. But here's the payoff—the older man is much less likely to prematurely ejaculate and will also take longer to ejaculate, progressing more slowly than the younger man through the stages of sexual response. Start thinking quality, not quantity, and you'll get the idea. As I said earlier, younger, single males are kind of like starving wolves roaming the forest. Even before they've finished eating, they're wondering where their next meal will come from, so they eat some more even when they're not hungry just in case the opportunity doesn't arise for a while!

What changes with age in a woman's sexual response?

Women who are postmenopausal tend to have lower levels of estrogen that can result in both a reduction of vaginal lubrication and taking a longer time for vaginal lubrication to occur. These changes, in addition to vaginal tissue losing tone, can cause uncomfortable or painful intercourse. Women can help to alleviate this situation by using some over-the-counter vaginal cream or lubrication. A woman's libido or sex drive may also diminish as she ages, and although ongoing research continues to examine ways to restore this drive, devices like the testosterone patch have produced inconsistent results.

What's the main reason for an older person not to have sex?

When asked the same question in 1974, famous sexologist Dr. Alex Comfort responded, "Old folks stop having sex for the same reason that they stop riding a bicycle—general infirmity (poor health), thinking it looks ridiculous, or no bicycle." Obviously, a person who is sick or infirm will have a much lower interest in sex than someone who is very healthy, and some individuals might simply be physically unable to have an active sex life.

Age can have a less than flattering effect on the body and so some individuals, particularly women, grow to feel very embarrassed and self-conscious about themselves, thus inhibiting sexual contact. In addition, society has conditioned older men and women to feel that they shouldn't even be having sexual thoughts, never mind sexual contact, and some individuals buy into this unfortunate ageist fallacy.

Don't forget that females live longer than males, so sooner or later older heterosexual women will find it difficult to find partners. By the age of eighty-five, women outnumber men by over two to one, and so partners are at a premium. Being a healthy, single, older male in assisted living is a hot ticket and will probably result in crazy action.

When do people stop being interested in sex?

For men, it's when they're dead. Men in particular tend to maintain an interest in sexual activity well into their later years, and if they are healthy will continue to be sexually active. Because men tend to die at a younger age than women, heterosexual older men tend to have little difficulty finding female partners. Women can also maintain a healthy interest in sex, although as they move through menopause, hormonal shifts often dull their sexual appetite. More research is being performed on older female sexuality and products such as a testosterone cream and testosterone patches exist in an attempt to kick-start the faltering libido. There are also fewer male partners available to older heterosexual women, so regardless of their libido, sexual outlets become more limited as women age. Having said that, there are many mature women who continue to enjoy active and satisfying sexual intimacy in their golden years.

PART FOUR

Our Sexual History

Early Influences

You have to wonder how we got so screwed up about sex. We can probably begin by blaming my English ancestors for shipping those Puritans to America four hundred years ago. The English certainly didn't want to keep those killjoys, and now Americans are stuck with their uncomfortable legacy. At the time of the early English settlement, the Puritan immigrants passed a series of laws that have since become known as the "sodomy laws." These sanctioned sexual intercourse as a behavior that could only occur during a marriage for the sole purpose of procreation. Hence, any sexual behavior that could not result in pregnancy was strictly forbidden. So let's think, what does that rule out? Oral sex, anal sex, and the solo sin of masturbation.

Strangely enough, because traveling was often difficult in the early days of settlement, on some occasions, a young man courting his sweetheart would be permitted to sleep in the same bed as her. Very liberal, you say? Well, not quite. First the couple would usually be fully clothed and wrapped in blankets (bundled up), and a plank or board, known as a bundling board, was placed between the couple. On some occasions a bundling bag would be used to further confine the suitor's movements, and quite often, because of a shortage of beds, the young woman's parents would sleep next to her. There's a libido killer!

What's truly amazing is that these so-called sodomy laws remained on the legislative books of nearly all states in some form until the Supreme Court effectively ruled against the laws in 2003. Just for your information, if you've ever had oral or anal sex in any of the following states prior to 2003 then you could have turned yourself in for a brief prison sentence. In Florida, you would've been charged with "unnatural and lascivious acts" and received sixty days in jail; in Louisiana, the same charge was a "crime against nature" with a possible five-year sentence; in Mississippi, you'd have received ten years for "unnatural intercourse"; and my very favorite crime description is "buggery" in South Carolina, which would have earned you five years in the big house. It's OK, relax, the sentences aren't retroactive!

Why are so many people so freaked out about sex today?

There's no question that some people have a really difficult time with sex and much of the difficulty dates back to our Puritan beginnings. However, a more recent legacy can be found in the works of nineteenth-century medical, religious, and academic "experts" who were only too eager to promote their bizarre ideas and pollute our psyches with negative misinformation.

For example, Sylvester Graham, a Presbyterian minister, believed that when a man ejaculated he lost the equivalent of forty ounces of blood, placing a great strain on his body. Graham recommended that a man ejaculate a maximum of twelve times each year! I have this visual of a guy who's already run through his twelve by February, and there he is, erection in hand, waiting for some type of apocalyptic moment as he nervously gives himself one last tug!

By the way, Sylvester Graham was the inventor of Graham crackers. Sylvester's contemporary, John Kellogg, in addition to being a developer of breakfast fodder, was another purveyor of misinformation. He believed that married couples should remain celibate after having children and gleefully described a man's erection as a "flagpole on your grave." Kellogg believed that bland foods would do much to promote abstinence, of which he was a big advocate.

What about the idea that women are less interested in sex?

These nineteenth-century experts did much to reinforce the double standard that still exists today—the concept that women have less interest in sex than men. Ironically, these mistaken medical men probably provided more sexual satisfaction for these "disinterested women" than their husbands.

At the turn of the twentieth century large proportions of women were being treated by doctors on a regular basis for a condition known as "hysteria." The remarkable treatment comprised a vulval massage, with doctors marveling how the women responded to the treatment with moans of "pain," with many rocking and shaking the treatment table, such was the intensity of their response. So while men were being told to eschew sexual contact, women were visiting their local, friendly masturbator—I mean doctor—for a quick rubdown. How sweet is that, and who was getting the better deal?

Another "expert," an English doctor called William Acton, instructed women to lie as still as possible during intercourse as any movement might interfere with conception, and unnecessary writhing was just plain undignified. Acton believed that a woman would simply endure intercourse in order to please her husband and have a family. If only he knew that she was climaxing once a week at the doctor's office. The irony is priceless.

More Recent Sexual Influences in America

How did World War II influence sexual mores?

World War II (1939–1945) had an immense influence on American sexual mores. Because the men were away fighting the war, women were forced to take their places in the factories, offices, and stores throughout the land. This shift pulled women out of the home in vast numbers, and to a great extent, many never went back, providing the impetus for a never before seen level of independence to be achieved decades later. This change in social roles afforded women the opportunity to enjoy a broader perspective on life, a perspective that inevitably included greater sexual activity. The men who went to war experienced new places, new customs, and to a great extent a freedom certainly not present in the United States at that time. The female movie star was a brand-new phenomenon, and the very first pin-up girl, Betty Grable, adorned many a GI's wall.

The American GI was a novelty in countries that had seen few Americans up close and personal. In England, where thousands of American servicemen were gathering for the D-Day invasion, their classy uniforms, better pay, and access to foods not seen for years led the jealous English military (including my dad!) to moan that there were three things wrong with American GIs: "they're overpaid, oversexed, and over here!"

In fact, American servicemen were so successful at "fraternizing" with the locals that as many as 20 percent may have contracted an infection of a sexual nature! At war's end, to deal with the huge influx of military personnel returning to the States with the gift that keeps on giving, special clinics were set up to handle the epidemic. American servicemen might have been coming home, but home would never be the same again for men and women alike.

Kinsey, Masters and Johnson—who were these guys?

In the late 1940s, a professor of zoology at Indiana University named Alfred Kinsey was asked to teach a course on human sexuality. He soon discovered that there was very little research performed on American sexual behavior. Inspired, he put together a team of research assistants, developed a highly complicated and innovative coding system, and proceeded to collect the most thorough information on sexual behavior ever generated. When his volumes were published in 1948 and 1953, the response to his work was less than enthusiastic. *The New York Times* refused to publish book reviews and a congressional subcommittee voiced concern that Kinsey's work would threaten the fabric of the American family. Not helping the cause was the rumor that Kinsey encouraged his research team to swap sexual partners, become more experienced sexually, and that Kinsey himself experimented with same-gender sex. Personally, I think Kinsey's finding that women were more likely to orgasm through masturbation than through penis-vagina intercourse was his downfall. Who's going to embrace research that makes the penis powerless?

Masters and Johnson were famous for observing thousands of orgasms in a laboratory setting. What's up with that? They were a husband-and-wife team who were trying to document how the body responds to sexual stimulation. Although some of you might think that the 1960s was the Dark Ages, the fact that only forty years ago science couldn't readily explain human sexual response is astonishing. "But why do we care?" you ask. Because when your body finally betrays you and lets you down at a very inopportune moment (we call that sexual dysfunction) you need to know how to fix the problem. All those erectile dysfunction ads you see on television couldn't exist without the work of Masters and Johnson forty years ago. So if you're getting a little chemical help with that erection, say a silent prayer of gratitude to this team of researchers. They watched so we could learn!

Were the "swinging sixties" really a sexual revolution?

Great question. Compared to the rather formal and staid decade of the fifties, I strongly believe that a social revolution occurred during the following decade. The sixties were certainly tempestuous times, where fashions and hairstyles pushed the envelope, adventurous musical sounds personified by Woodstock replaced the elevator music masquerading as entertainment, the Vietnam War galvanized an exuberant youth into rebellion, and perhaps the most significant influence on sexual behavior of the century was released into this bubbling cauldron—the pill. For the very first time in the history of the world, women would be able to have sexual intercourse and not fear pregnancy.

Certainly, the early twentieth century was not very accepting of single mothers, and my guess would be that although women of this time were just as interested in sex as their contemporaries today, the ever present fear of pregnancy and its accompanying social disgrace was enough to temper the ardor of many a young woman. The pill represented a means of achieving sexual freedom, and was introduced into a decade that was more than ready to embrace it. The sexual world would be changed forever.

Do presidents like sex?

In more recent years, America's leaders have tried to set our sexual ship of state on some type of course, often erratic and always inconsistent. President Reagan attempted to enforce what became known as the "squeal rules," in which females who were minors would have to obtain written parental consent before they could obtain contraception. President Reagan felt this law would bring the American family closer together. Right. "Oh Dad, Danny and I are going up to the lake this evening. There's a good chance we're going to have sex, so could I get a letter from you so I can get some contraception?" "Of course, Lori, no problem. Just make sure Danny gets some condoms too because you don't want to get a bad case of chlamydia, now do you? Pass the salt, please."

President Clinton gave the country an unexpected primer on the definition of sex, the meaning of oral sex, and a thousand and one things you can do with a cigar. This is the same president, by the way, who asked for his surgeon general's resignation after she suggested that masturbation might be a good way to go, given the number of diseases out there. The nerve of the woman!

Perhaps President Bush II was still smarting over Bill Clinton's national sex education lessons when he came to power, because that can be the only logical reason why he has allowed his abstinence-until-marriage obsession to override sheer common sense, not to mention a boatload of scientific evidence to the contrary. In 2007 the federal government recommended that the concept of abstinence-until-marriage should be expanded to encourage unmarried folks up to the age of twenty-nine to remain abstinent. That should work.

How did this whole abstinence-only-until-marriage education thing get started?

Once upon a time, there was a group of very religious men who also happened to be politicians of influence—like the president and his friends. They decided that despite the best available scientific evidence, the single most effective way to reduce adolescent sexual activity was to have the schools of our nation teach only about abstinence. The politicians of influence were able to accomplish this quite easily by creating a situation where unless states agreed, they would not receive approximately two million dollars a year in federal funding. This type of arrangement is most commonly known as *blackmail*, but then maybe I've seen too many episodes of *Law & Order*.

So, does abstinence-only-until-marriage education actually work?

There is no research data on this planet to support the theory that telling adolescents never to have sex really works. But then, when did a one-size-fits-all solution solve any problem? Mathematica Policy Research, Inc., a prestigious research organization based in Princeton, New Jersey, published the most thorough and well-documented evaluation of abstinence-only programs in 2007, and reported that these programs were ineffective. Under any other administration, such findings would be the death knell for abstinence-only education. Don't hold your breath!

This may sound like a dumb question, but what is abstinence?

Actually, that's a very smart question, because if we reverse it to read, "What is sex?" we have the same difficulty. The folks who pushed the abstinence-only education, in their infinite wisdom, chose not to define what abstinence is, because if they did that, they might have had to discuss nonprocreative sexual behavior like oral sex and anal sex, to say nothing of masturbation. If I have massive amounts of cunnilingus (oral-vaginal) sex, am I still abstinent? If a person fellates (oral-penis) a hundred penises a week, is he/she still abstinent? The advocates of abstinence-only education initially defined sex so narrowly that "other activities" were barely considered, despite scientific data suggesting that adolescents are way more likely to be putting their mouths on things than experiencing coitus (penis-vagina intercourse).

So Where Do We Go from Here? A Note to the Reader

Acknowledging your sexual ignorance is not to blame you for what you don't know—it's not your fault. It has everything to do with our culture's inability to accept and incorporate human sexuality as an important part of our education. Despite the fact that we're inundated with unfiltered, unscreened sexual messaging, our country's leaders and educators have been too busy bickering about the "correct" approach to actually provide any meaningful direction.

In the United States, sexual behavior today, or rather the fallout from sexual behavior, is viewed by many as a moral issue. In other Western industrialized nations, populations have seemingly escaped the "sex equals guilt and shame" equation (the English, of course, live sex-guilt free because they shipped those sanctimonious, religious immigrants over here 260 years ago). The negative consequences of sexual behavior are viewed not as moral slips, but rather as public health problems that deserve a public health response—prevention and treatment, *without* the moralistic sermon!

If you think I'm making this up, check out the proportion of unintended pregnancy and abortion rates among populations in Europe versus the United States. In fact, our closest neighbor to the north, Canada, has a teen unintended pregnancy rate that is dwarfed by ours. How can that be? Do the Canadian border guards force a condom on you as you cross to buy your cheap medication? How is it that the Netherlands, probably the most liberal nation on the planet, has the lowest teenage pregnancy rates of pretty much any country in the world, and as a result, has made abortion an afterthought? The huge difference is that other countries treat human sexuality as a *regular part* of a person's life and existence. And although their citizens are exposed to the same sexualizing influences as their peers in America, they are also provided with a much more stabilizing and balanced educational environment.

This book hasn't spent much time discussing abstinence, but in reality, sexual intercourse isn't a mandatory activity for anyone. You don't have to have sex with everyone you're seeing, and even if you have been sexually active with your last partner, that doesn't necessarily mean you have to be with the next. You do have choices, so exercise them.

The fact that so many young women over the years have described how uncomfortable they feel about sex and how they really don't enjoy it that much is a red flag to me. When I ask the women why they're having sex if they don't feel good about it, the inevitable answer is "because my boyfriend wants to." I repeat, sex is not mandatory. I know the pressures to be sexually active are intense for both women *and* men, but I'd encourage you to examine your own feelings about each situation and don't just follow the path of least resistance.

If you do choose to be sexually active, then expect to get an STI, and if you're straight, expect to get someone pregnant or become pregnant! This rather grim prediction is a cue for you to take adequate precautions. ALWAYS use a condom plus any other legitimate contraceptive device discussed earlier. If you have a partner who is reluctant or even unwilling to use protection, then tell him or her to get lost. You have to protect yourself; no one else is going to do it for you. Sex on your terms or not at all.

So now that you've read the wild and weird things in this book, and hopefully had some questions answered, what should you take away from the experience, other than loads of laughs? Although I always receive a lot of questions about sexual anatomy and response—things like penis size, vaginal lubrication, clitoral stimulation, oral sex, multiple orgasms and so on, the single largest category of items relates to communication—particularly between the sexes. The understanding between men and women in sexual situations seems tenuous at best, and for many, nonexistent.

Although talking about sex can be excruciatingly difficult and embarrassing, you *have* to communicate more. Communication will help you in so many ways, from deciding whether or not you even want to have sex, to negotiating condom use that can prevent pregnancy, HIV, and STI transmission; decrease the likelihood of date rape; and simply make you feel a lot closer to your partner. There's simply no downside to communication, and yet most of us find it so difficult. Now that you've become a *sexpert,* I can only hope you're better prepared to face the world of human sexuality with confidence and, of course, a smile on your face.

Acknowledgments

Writing a book can be a study in solitude, but the entire process is really something that can't be effectively accomplished without the help of some very important people. I'm so grateful to my literary agents Rafe Sagalyn and Bridget Wagner of the Sagalyn Agency for their vision, insight, support, and unfailing enthusiasm. This project would never have been developed without you. I'd also like to thank Patrick Price, my editor at Simon Spotlight Entertainment, for having the courage to run with a book like this and helping to keep me in check . . . sort of! My wife and partner in crime, Anne, was a terrific reader and editor and I can't thank her enough for helping me with the content and having the courage to tell me when I was crossing the line! I had the good fortune to work with an outstanding research assistant in Stacy Glantz—thanks for delving into the deep pools of sexual weirdness; I'm sure you made your parents proud!

Finally, I'd like to thank a particularly large group of people without whom this book would have had a lot of empty pages—the 16,000 or more students who have participated in my sexuality class (HLTH 377) since 1984 at the University of Maryland. The wonder of my job has been that four times a year, for as long as I can remember, I've met a new group of enthusiastic, motivated, often crazy students who were more than willing participants on my semester's journey through the world of human sexuality. You energized me, you shocked me, you always made me laugh and, ultimately, you taught me much more than I could ever teach you. And now your questions are recorded for all to see in the pages of this book. You know who you are—thanks for your enthusiasm and energy. You made my job a breeze.

D
R

R
O
B
I
N

S
A
W
Y
E
R

About the Author

ROBIN SAWYER was born and raised in England. He was a high school teacher before coming to the United States in 1974, where he accepted a soccer scholarship at George Mason University. He completed his master's degree at the University of Virginia and doctorate at the University of Maryland.

Robin has been a faculty member at the University of Maryland since 1984, and speaks extensively around the country on human sexuality, working particularly closely with university athletes on the issue of date rape and sexual assault.

He currently lives in Columbia, Maryland, with his wife, Anne, also a sexuality educator, where they have raised their four daughters, Katherine, Emily, Meg, and Gillian.